White Coat Without Borders

The Definitive Step-by-Step Guide for International Medical Graduates to Become U.S. Physicians

SOPHIA KANGARLU

MD, FACP, CHCQM, MBA, FABQAURP.

ISBN: 9798243196918 (Paperback)

Library of Congress Control Number: 2026900473

Any references to historical events, real people, or real places are used fictitiously. Names, characters, and places are products of the author's imagination.

First printing edition 2026.

Disclaimer

The information provided in this book, *From Abroad to MD: A Complete Guide for International Medical Graduates in the U.S.*, is for educational and informational purposes only. While every effort has been made to ensure the accuracy, completeness, and reliability of the content, the author and publisher make no representations or warranties of any kind, express or implied, regarding the accuracy or applicability of the information contained herein.

The guidance, examples, and resources provided reflect general knowledge and publicly available information as of the time of publication. Rules, regulations, and procedures related to U.S. medical licensing, residency applications, visas, and professional certification change frequently. Readers are encouraged to verify details with official sources before making any decisions.

This book does not constitute legal, immigration, or professional advice. The author and publisher shall not be liable for any loss or damages, direct or indirect, arising from the use or misuse of the information contained in this publication.

All trademarks, logos, and names of organizations mentioned in this book are the property of their respective owners and are used for identification purposes only.

Contents

Disclaimer 4

Introduction: The IMG Journey 6

Chapter 1: Understanding the U.S. Medical System 19

Chapter 2: Preparing Before Arrival 37

Chapter 3: First Steps in the U.S. 63

Chapter 4: The USMLE Roadmap 84

Chapter 5: Clinical Experience in the U.S. 108

Chapter 6: Research and Publications 134

Chapter 7: Applying to Residency Programs 156

Chapter 8: The Interview Process 182

Chapter 9: Residency Life as an IMG 202

Chapter 10: Beyond Residency - Fellowships and Practice 217

Chapter 11: Transitioning from Practicing Physician Abroad to U.S. Trainee 233

Chapter 12: Specialty Choice for Experienced Physicians 243

Chapter 13: Leveraging International Experience in the Residency Match 255

Chapter 14: Life After Residency for Experienced IMGs 266

Introduction:

The IMG Journey

When you land in the United States as an international medical graduate (IMG), you carry more than a suitcase. You carry years of training, sleepless nights, countless exams, and the dream of becoming a physician who heals lives across borders. But as many discover quickly, stepping onto U.S. soil is only the beginning of another journey - a journey just as demanding and transformative as medical school itself.

This book is written for you: the foreign medical graduate (FMG) or international medical graduate (IMG) who aspires to practice medicine in the U.S. Whether you have just arrived, are preparing to move, or are already knee-deep in board exams, clinical rotations, and residency applications, this book will serve as a roadmap, companion, and guide.

A Glimpse into the IMG Experience

Consider this composite story, drawn from the lives of many IMGs:

Anita, a physician trained in India, dreamed of practicing internal medicine in the U.S. She had excelled in her MBBS program, completed an internship, and even gained clinical experience at a well-respected hospital in her hometown.

But upon arriving in New York, she quickly realized that her medical degree, while valuable, wasn't enough to walk into a hospital as a doctor. She needed to pass the U.S. licensing exams, gain clinical experience in the U.S., and navigate the daunting process of applying for residency.

She faced moments of doubt: Should she spend her limited savings on a prep course or hold onto the money for rent? Could she really compete with U.S. medical graduates who already knew the system? And what if she failed an exam?

Yet Anita persisted. She leaned on IMG networks, studied late nights with UWorld and First Aid, volunteered in hospitals, and slowly built her application. Years later, she matched into a residency program in internal medicine. Today, she's a practicing physician in Chicago, mentoring the next generation of IMGs.

This story is not unusual. It reflects the resilience, grit, and courage of thousands of IMGs who every year cross oceans - literally and figuratively - to build their future in American medicine.

Why IMGs Matter in U.S. Healthcare

The U.S. healthcare system depends on international medical graduates more than many realize. According to the ECFMG (Educational Commission for Foreign Medical Graduates), around one in four practicing physicians in the United States is an IMG.

That means if you've visited a hospital in the U.S., chances are you've been treated by an IMG.

Why are IMGs so vital?

Physician shortages. The U.S. faces a looming physician shortage, with estimates suggesting a gap of more than 124,000 doctors by 2034. IMGs help fill critical shortages, especially in primary care, internal medicine, and underserved rural and urban communities.

Diversity and cultural competence. IMGs bring linguistic skills, cultural understanding, and a global perspective to healthcare. In an increasingly diverse U.S. population, patients often feel more comfortable with physicians who share their cultural background or speak their language.

Dedication and perseverance. The very act of navigating the U.S. medical system as an IMG requires determination, adaptability, and resilience - the same qualities that make exceptional physicians.

Without IMGs, many communities would lack adequate healthcare access. This book acknowledges not just your struggle, but your importance to the American healthcare landscape.

The IMG Journey: What Lies Ahead

Every IMG's path is different, but most face similar milestones. Broadly, your journey can be broken down into five stages:

Arrival: Settling into U.S. life - finding housing, managing finances, overcoming culture shock, and building a support system.

Exams: Preparing for and passing the United States Medical Licensing Examination (USMLE) steps - arguably the most defining part of the IMG journey.

Medical school pathways (if needed): Some IMGs choose additional U.S. education, such as an MPH, MS, or even repeating part of medical school, to strengthen their residency applications.

Residency: Applying to and matching with a U.S. residency program, which is the gateway to medical practice.

Integration: Adjusting to residency life, navigating visas and work challenges, and ultimately thriving as a physician in the U.S.

This book will walk you through each of these phases, providing both practical advice (how to apply for observerships, which visa options exist) and emotional support (how to deal with rejection, isolation, and burnout).

What Makes the IMG Journey Unique

For U.S. medical graduates, the path is straightforward: medical school → USMLE exams → residency. For IMGs, the path is rarely linear. You face additional hurdles. Some of these include:

Proving your credentials are valid.

Understanding a new healthcare culture.

Learning U.S.-style communication with patients.

Navigating immigration laws and visa restrictions.

Competing for limited residency spots as an international applicant.

But with every challenge comes opportunity. Many IMGs develop stronger adaptability, cultural awareness, and problem-solving skills simply by navigating this process. These qualities often make them stand out in residency programs and beyond.

Over the years, I've seen countless IMGs succeed, and countless others give up. Some drop out because the process seems too complicated. Others lose hope after one rejection. Too many waste time and money on misinformation, or feel they have to figure it all out alone.

This book is written with the intention to change that.

It's practical. You'll find checklists, timelines, and strategies that you can apply immediately.

It's realistic. I won't sugarcoat the challenges. The road is hard, and not everyone succeeds on the first try. But knowing the obstacles ahead prepares you to overcome them.

It's inspiring. Alongside practical advice, you'll read stories of IMGs who have walked this path, stumbled, and risen stronger.

My goal is simple: to help you not just survive this journey, but thrive.

How This Book Is Structured

The chapters are organized to follow your journey step by step:

Chapter 1 explains the U.S. medical system and how it differs from your home country.

Chapter 2 guides you through preparation before you even arrive.

Chapter 3 focuses on your first steps in the U.S. - from cultural adaptation to daily logistics.

Chapter 4 maps out the USMLE exams with strategies and resources.

Chapter 5 shows how to gain U.S. clinical experience and secure strong letters of recommendation.

Chapter 6 covers research and publications.

Chapter 7 and 8 help you navigate the residency application and interview process.

Chapter 9 and 10 explore residency life, fellowships, and career pathways after training.

Chapters 11 to 14 focus on MD doctors who have already completed their specialization and want to come to the US for residency.

Think of this book as both a manual and a companion, something you'll return to whenever you hit a roadblock.

A Word of Encouragement

Becoming a doctor in the U.S. as an IMG is not just about passing exams or landing a residency. It's about perseverance, adaptability, and courage. You will face moments of doubt - nights where the textbooks blur before your eyes, or mornings when rejection letters make you question your worth.

But remember this: you are not alone. Thousands have walked this path before you. They too felt lost, uncertain, and overwhelmed. And yet, many found their way to white coats, stethoscopes, and the honor of serving patients in the U.S.

If you are holding this book, you already have what it takes - the determination to keep going.

From Abroad to MD is more than a how-to guide. It's a roadmap, a mentor, and at times, a voice reminding you that your dream is possible. By the end of this book, you'll not only understand the steps ahead but also feel empowered to take them, confidently, strategically, and with resilience.

So, welcome to the journey. It won't be easy. But it will be worth it.

Consider this composite story, drawn from the lives of many IMGs:

Anita, a physician trained in India, dreamed of practicing internal medicine in the U.S. She had excelled in her MBBS program, completed an internship, and even gained clinical experience at a well-respected hospital in her hometown.

But upon arriving in New York, she quickly realized that her medical degree, while valuable, wasn't enough to walk into a hospital as a doctor. She needed to pass the U.S. licensing exams, gain clinical experience in the U.S., and navigate the daunting process of applying for residency.

She faced moments of doubt: Should she spend her limited savings on a prep course or hold onto the money for rent? Could she really compete with U.S. medical graduates who already knew the system? And what if she failed an exam?

Yet Anita persisted. She leaned on IMG networks, studied late nights with UWorld and First Aid, volunteered in hospitals, and slowly built her application. Years later, she matched into a residency program in internal medicine. Today, she's a practicing physician in Chicago, mentoring the next generation of IMGs.

This story is not unusual. It reflects the resilience, grit, and courage of thousands of IMGs who every year cross oceans - literally and figuratively - to build their future in American medicine.

Why IMGs Matter in U.S. Healthcare

The U.S. healthcare system depends on international medical graduates more than many realize. According to the ECFMG (Educational Commission for Foreign Medical Graduates), around one in four practicing physicians in the United States is an IMG.

That means if you've visited a hospital in the U.S., chances are you've been treated by an IMG.

Why are IMGs so vital?

Physician shortages. The U.S. faces a looming physician shortage, with estimates suggesting a gap of more than 124,000 doctors by 2034. IMGs help fill critical shortages, especially in primary care, internal medicine, and underserved rural and urban communities.

Diversity and cultural competence. IMGs bring linguistic skills, cultural understanding, and a global perspective to healthcare. In an increasingly diverse U.S. population, patients often feel more comfortable with physicians who share their cultural background or speak their language.

Dedication and perseverance. The very act of navigating the U.S. medical system as an IMG requires determination, adaptability, and resilience - the same qualities that make exceptional physicians.

Without IMGs, many communities would lack adequate healthcare access. This book acknowledges not just your struggle, but your importance to the American healthcare landscape.

The IMG Journey: What Lies Ahead

Every IMG's path is different, but most face similar milestones. Broadly, your journey can be broken down into five stages:

Arrival: Settling into U.S. life - finding housing, managing finances, overcoming culture shock, and building a support system.

Exams: Preparing for and passing the United States Medical Licensing Examination (USMLE) steps - arguably the most defining part of the IMG journey.

Medical school pathways (if needed): Some IMGs choose additional U.S. education, such as an MPH, MS, or even repeating part of medical school, to strengthen their residency applications.

Residency: Applying to and matching with a U.S. residency program, which is the gateway to medical practice.

Integration: Adjusting to residency life, navigating visas and work challenges, and ultimately thriving as a physician in the U.S.

This book will walk you through each of these phases, providing both practical advice (how to apply for observerships, which visa options exist) and emotional support (how to deal with rejection, isolation, and burnout).

What Makes the IMG Journey Unique

For U.S. medical graduates, the path is straightforward: medical school → USMLE exams → residency. For IMGs, the path is rarely linear. You face additional hurdles. Some of these include:

Proving your credentials are valid.

Understanding a new healthcare culture.

Learning U.S.-style communication with patients.

Navigating immigration laws and visa restrictions.

Competing for limited residency spots as an international applicant.

But with every challenge comes opportunity. Many IMGs develop stronger adaptability, cultural awareness, and problem-solving skills simply by navigating this process. These qualities often make them stand out in residency programs and beyond.

Over the years, I've seen countless IMGs succeed, and countless others give up. Some drop out because the process seems too complicated. Others lose hope after one rejection. Too many waste time and money on misinformation, or feel they have to figure it all out alone.

This book is written with the intention to change that.

It's practical. You'll find checklists, timelines, and strategies that you can apply immediately.

It's realistic. I won't sugarcoat the challenges. The road is hard, and not everyone succeeds on the first try. But knowing the obstacles ahead prepares you to overcome them.

It's inspiring. Alongside practical advice, you'll read stories of IMGs who have walked this path, stumbled, and risen stronger.

My goal is simple: to help you not just survive this journey, but thrive.

How This Book Is Structured

The chapters are organized to follow your journey step by step:

Chapter 1 explains the U.S. medical system and how it differs from your home country.

Chapter 2 guides you through preparation before you even arrive.

Chapter 3 focuses on your first steps in the U.S. - from cultural adaptation to daily logistics.

Chapter 4 maps out the USMLE exams with strategies and resources.

Chapter 5 shows how to gain U.S. clinical experience and secure strong letters of recommendation.

Chapter 6 covers research and publications.

Chapter 7 and 8 help you navigate the residency application and interview process.

Chapter 9 and 10 explore residency life, fellowships, and career pathways after training.

Chapters 11 to 14 focus on MD doctors who have already completed their specialization and want to come to the US for residency.

Think of this book as both a manual and a companion, something you'll return to whenever you hit a roadblock.

A Word of Encouragement

Becoming a doctor in the U.S. as an IMG is not just about passing exams or landing a residency. It's about perseverance, adaptability, and courage. You will face moments of doubt - nights where the textbooks blur before your eyes, or mornings when rejection letters make you question your worth.

But remember this: you are not alone. Thousands have walked this path before you. They too felt lost, uncertain, and overwhelmed. And yet, many found their way to white coats, stethoscopes, and the honor of serving patients in the U.S.

If you are holding this book, you already have what it takes - the determination to keep going.

From Abroad to MD is more than a how-to guide. It's a roadmap, a mentor, and at times, a voice reminding you that your dream is possible. By the end of this book, you'll not only understand the steps ahead but also feel empowered to take them, confidently, strategically, and with resilience.

So, welcome to the journey. It won't be easy. But it will be worth it.

Chapter 1:
Understanding the U.S. Medical System

When international medical graduates (IMGs) arrive in the United States, one of the first challenges they encounter is understanding how the U.S. medical system functions.

This challenge is twofold: first, the structure of medical education and training is significantly different from that of many other countries; second, the healthcare delivery system itself, how patients receive care, how doctors practice, and how hospitals operate, is unique, complex, and often confusing even to U.S. citizens.

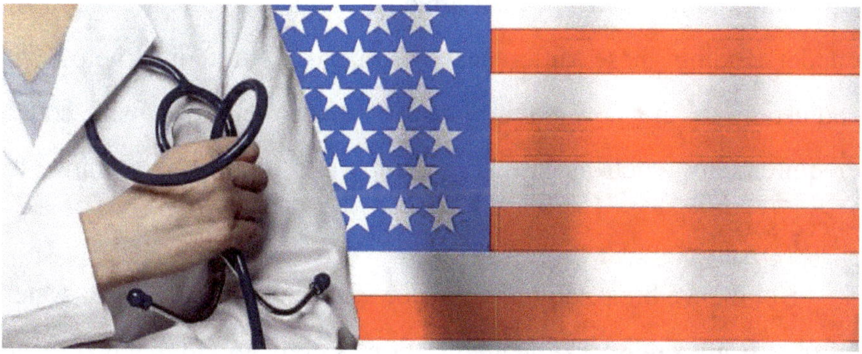

For IMGs, the journey to becoming a practicing physician in America requires not just passing exams, but also learning to navigate an entirely different medical culture.

This chapter provides a foundation: the differences between foreign and U.S. medical education, an overview of the healthcare system, the role of key accreditation bodies, and, finally, how IMGs fit into the U.S. medical workforce.

Key Differences Between U.S. and Foreign Medical Education Systems

Medical education is one of the most challenging and rewarding journeys in the world. No matter where it takes place, the ultimate goal is the same: to produce skilled, compassionate, and knowledgeable physicians who can care for patients safely and effectively.

But the path to becoming a doctor is not uniform across the globe. The structure, terminology, and expectations of medical education vary depending on geography, culture, and history.

For international medical graduates entering the U.S. system, understanding these differences is crucial. It not only helps with adjusting to the new environment, but also clarifies why certain requirements, such as licensing exams and additional training, are necessary.

Below, we break down the major ways in which the U.S. system differs from foreign medical education systems, and what that means for aspiring physicians.

Pathway to Medicine: Undergraduate vs. Graduate Entry Age

One of the most significant differences between the U.S. and many other countries is the point at which medical education begins.

In most of the world: Students enter medicine directly after high school.

- **India:** At around age 17 or 18, students who succeed in competitive entrance exams are admitted into the MBBS (Bachelor of Medicine, Bachelor of Surgery) program. This program usually lasts 5.5 years, including a one-year compulsory internship.
- **Europe:** Countries such as Germany, Italy, and France offer integrated six-year programs in which students study pre-clinical sciences and clinical subjects in one continuous stream.
- **Middle East and Africa:** Similar MBBS pathways exist, blending early science courses with clinical exposure in the later years.

However, in the U.S., medicine is not a direct-entry program. Instead, it is considered a graduate-level profession. Students must first complete a four-year undergraduate (bachelor's) degree, usually with a focus on science subjects such as biology, chemistry, or neuroscience. After that, they apply to medical school, which itself is another four years of training.

This distinction has practical consequences. U.S. medical graduates are typically older by the time they begin residency. Many are in their mid-twenties or later, while IMGs from direct-entry programs may already be qualified doctors, with an internship completed, by age 23 or 24.

Degrees Awarded

Another major source of confusion is the degree title itself.

Medical schools in the United States award either an MD (Doctor of Medicine) or a DO (Doctor of Osteopathic Medicine) degree. Both represent fully licensed physicians, though DOs receive additional training in osteopathic manipulative treatment and often emphasize holistic, patient-centered care.

In most other countries, the degree is usually the MBBS (Bachelor of Medicine, Bachelor of Surgery) or one of its variants (MBChB, BMBS). Despite the word *"bachelor"* in the title, this is a professional degree equivalent to the MD in terms of scope and recognition.

For patients, employers, and even residency program directors unfamiliar with global medical systems, the terminology can sometimes cause misunderstanding. An IMG with an MBBS may need to explain that their degree reflects the same level of medical training as an MD, not a lower-level qualification.

Curriculum and Teaching Style

The structure of the curriculum also differs significantly.

In U.S. medical schools, the first two years are largely classroom-based but incorporate modern teaching methods such as problem-based learning (PBL), team-based case discussions, and simulation labs. Students study anatomy, physiology, biochemistry, and pathology, but these subjects are taught alongside clinical skills and early patient interactions.

The final two years are spent in clinical clerkships, rotating through specialties such as internal medicine, surgery, pediatrics, psychiatry, obstetrics and gynecology, and family medicine. Students are assessed using standardized criteria to ensure uniform competency.

In most foreign systems, the first half of medical school is usually lecture-heavy and didactic, with a strong emphasis on theory and memorization. Students often spend two to three years focusing on pre-clinical sciences before stepping into a hospital ward.

Clinical rotations may begin later and vary widely in intensity depending on the institution. Some students gain extensive hands-on experience, while others primarily shadow senior doctors with limited direct patient responsibility.

This variation means that while many IMGs have excellent medical knowledge, they sometimes need additional supervised U.S. clinical experience, such as observerships or externships, to demonstrate their ability to function effectively within the American system of patient care.

Clinical Experience

Clinical exposure is one of the biggest differentiators between systems.

In the U.S., clerkships are standardized, carefully supervised, and competency-driven. Students are expected to take patient histories, perform physical examinations, and actively participate in patient care, all under the guidance of attending physicians and residents.

Additionally, each student rotates through a set of mandatory core specialties, ensuring broad exposure before residency.

In other countries, the level of clinical exposure often depends heavily on the medical college's resources and affiliated teaching hospitals. Some students graduate with a high degree of responsibility for patient care, particularly in countries with limited healthcare staff, while others may not receive the same depth of supervised training.

This inconsistency is one reason the U.S. places such strong emphasis on IMGs completing clinical observerships or externships in the U.S. prior to residency applications. These experiences allow program directors to assess how international graduates adapt to the expectations and workflow of American hospitals.

Licensing Examinations

Perhaps the most daunting difference for IMGs is the licensing examination structure.

In the U.S., all medical students must pass the United States Medical Licensing Examination (USMLE) series. This standardized system is designed to ensure that every physician, regardless of where they were trained, meets the same baseline of medical knowledge and clinical competence.

The USMLE consists of the following steps:

- **Step 1:** Focuses on basic sciences and is often regarded as one of the most challenging hurdles. It tests subjects such as anatomy, physiology, pharmacology, pathology, and microbiology, emphasizing the application of foundational science to clinical scenarios.
- **Step 2 CK (Clinical Knowledge):** Assesses the application of medical knowledge in clinical settings, including diagnosis, management, and patient care across a broad range of specialties.
- **Step 3:** Typically taken during or after residency, this exam evaluates readiness for independent medical practice.

In contrast, licensing structures in other countries vary widely. Some nations have their own standardized national exams, such as the PLAB in the United Kingdom, while others rely primarily on university-based assessments without a single centralized licensing system.

This makes the U.S. system uniquely rigorous and standardized. While it ensures uniformity and quality, it also creates a significant barrier for IMGs, who must pass the same exams as U.S. medical students to demonstrate equivalency. For many IMGs, preparing for and passing the USMLE exams represents the single most demanding challenge of their journey.

Postgraduate Training

Postgraduate training, what happens after medical school, also looks very different in the United States compared to many other countries.

In the U.S., residency training is highly structured, nationally standardized, and accredited by the Accreditation Council for Graduate Medical Education (ACGME). Residency programs typically last between three and seven years, depending on the specialty.

Entry into residency is extremely competitive and is managed through the National Resident Matching Program (NRMP), a centralized matching system that pairs applicants with residency programs based on ranked preferences from both sides.

Residents in the U.S. are considered full members of the healthcare team. From the beginning of training, they assume real clinical responsibilities, with increasing autonomy under supervision as they progress through the program.

In many other countries, graduates may work as “house officers,” “junior doctors,” or medical officers before entering formal specialty training. In some systems, postgraduate training is less standardized, and the quality of training may depend heavily on the institution, region, or availability of senior supervision.

In certain countries, physicians may practice independently in limited roles without completing a structured residency program equivalent to U.S. standards.

For IMGs, this difference has significant implications. Even physicians who have practiced independently abroad are generally required to complete a full U.S. residency program in order to obtain licensure and practice independently in the United States.

Although the ultimate goal of medical education worldwide is the same, the pathway, structure, and expectations surrounding postgraduate training differ dramatically. Understanding this reality early helps IMGs align expectations and prepare mentally for retraining within a new system.

U.S. Healthcare System Overview

The United States healthcare system is one of the most complex and distinctive in the world. For international medical graduates, adjusting to its structure can feel overwhelming, particularly when compared to the more centralized and uniform healthcare systems found in countries such as the United Kingdom, Canada, or many parts of Europe.

While the U.S. system is often criticized for its cost and inequities, it is also known for innovation, advanced technology, and a strong emphasis on patient-centered care.

For IMGs preparing to train and practice in America, understanding how care is organized, delivered, and financed is not merely an academic exercise, it is essential for providing safe, effective, and ethical care.

This section explores the major components of the U.S. healthcare system, its accreditation structures, and the roles IMGs play within it.

Insurance-Based System

One of the defining features of U.S. healthcare is its multi-payer insurance model, which distinguishes it from countries with nationalized or single-payer systems. Rather than universal coverage provided by the government, Americans obtain healthcare through a combination of private and public insurance programs.

Private Insurance

Nearly half of all Americans receive health insurance through their employer. Employers contract with private insurance companies, and employees typically share the cost through payroll deductions.

Coverage varies widely depending on the plan. Some policies offer generous benefits, while others require high deductibles, copayments, and coinsurance.

For IMGs, this can be surprising. In countries with nationalized healthcare systems, patients rarely consider whether they can afford a diagnostic test or procedure. In the U.S., however, even insured patients may hesitate to pursue recommended care because of out-of-pocket costs.

Example: A patient with chest pain may delay seeing a cardiologist due to high copayments, potentially resulting in disease progression. IMGs often notice how financial considerations influence medical decision-making in ways they may not have encountered in their home countries.

Public Insurance

Two major government-sponsored programs provide coverage for specific populations:

1. **Medicare:** A federal program primarily serving individuals aged 65 and older, as well as certain younger patients with disabilities or end-stage renal disease. Medicare is divided into several parts:
    a. Part A: Hospital insurance
    b. Part B: Medical insurance for outpatient care
    c. Part C: Medicare Advantage plans administered by private insurers
    d. Part D: Prescription drug coverage
2. **Medicaid:** A joint federal and state program designed for low-income individuals and families. Eligibility criteria and covered services vary by state, meaning that access to care can differ significantly across the country.

The Uninsured

Despite the availability of public and private insurance options, millions of Americans remain uninsured. These individuals often delay preventive care and rely heavily on emergency departments or community clinics.

As a result, IMGs working in U.S. hospitals frequently encounter patients presenting with advanced disease due to lack of access to earlier care.

By contrast, in Canada's single-payer system, every citizen has coverage. Emergency departments there tend to see fewer patients seeking care for chronic conditions that could have been managed earlier in primary care settings.

The absence of universal healthcare coverage remains one of the most significant challenges within the U.S. system. IMGs must learn to navigate the ethical and practical realities of caring for patients who may be unable to afford recommended treatments.

Patient-Centered Care

A cornerstone of modern U.S. medicine is the emphasis on patient-centered care. This philosophy requires that patients actively participate in their healthcare decisions, guided-but not dictated-by their physicians.

Shared Decision-Making

Unlike in more paternalistic systems, where doctors make decisions on behalf of patients, U.S. physicians are expected to explain options, risks, and benefits while respecting patient preferences.

Example: A U.S. oncologist may spend significant time discussing the pros and cons of chemotherapy versus palliative care, allowing the patient and their family to decide based on values and quality-of-life considerations.

For IMGs trained in systems where physician authority is rarely questioned, this adjustment can be profound. Patients in the U.S. often arrive well-informed, having researched their conditions online, and expect to voice opinions about their treatment.

Informed Consent and Autonomy

Legal frameworks in the U.S. emphasize autonomy and require thorough informed consent. Before a surgery, for instance, patients must be given clear explanations of risks, alternatives, and expected outcomes. Failing to do so can have legal consequences.

Cultural Sensitivity

The U.S. is an incredibly diverse nation, with patients from every cultural, religious, and linguistic background. Physicians must demonstrate cultural competence, ensuring that care is respectful and responsive to cultural health beliefs and practices.

For IMGs, this environment can be both challenging and rewarding. Their multilingual skills and cross-cultural backgrounds often make them particularly effective in connecting with diverse patient populations.

Interprofessional Collaboration

The U.S. healthcare system strongly emphasizes team-based care. Physicians rarely work in isolation and are instead part of interprofessional teams designed to improve patient outcomes.

Key Members of the Team

- **Nurses and Nurse Practitioners (NPs):** NPs can diagnose, prescribe medications, and manage chronic conditions independently in many states.
- **Physician Assistants (PAs):** Work under physician supervision but perform many of the same duties, including examinations, diagnosis, and prescribing.
- **Pharmacists:** Play an active role in medication management, patient counseling, and safety checks.
- **Social Workers:** Assist with social determinants of health, such as housing, financial barriers, and mental health support.
- **Physical and Occupational Therapists:** Aid in rehabilitation and functional recovery.

For IMGs, this team-based approach may initially feel unfamiliar. In some countries, physicians handle most responsibilities without significant input from other professionals. Learning to respect and coordinate with these roles is crucial for success in U.S. residency and practice.

Technology and Documentation

Another defining feature of U.S. healthcare is its reliance on technology, particularly Electronic Health Records (EHRs).

Electronic Health Records

Nearly all hospitals and clinics in the U.S. now use EHRs, which serve multiple purposes:

- Clinical documentation for continuity of care
- Billing and coding for insurance reimbursement
- Legal protection in case of disputes
- Quality reporting to meet regulatory requirements

For IMGs unfamiliar with EHRs, the steep learning curve can be overwhelming. Residents often find themselves spending as much, or more, time on documentation as on direct patient care.

Other Technologies

The U.S. system is also notable for its adoption of advanced medical technologies, from robotic surgery to telemedicine platforms. While these innovations improve care, they also increase costs and sometimes widen disparities, as not all patients can access the latest treatments.

Accreditation Bodies in the U.S.

The U.S. medical system is heavily regulated to ensure consistency, safety, and quality. Accreditation bodies govern every stage of a physician's training, and IMGs must understand their roles.

LCME – Liaison Committee on Medical Education

The LCME accredits MD-granting medical schools in the U.S. and Canada. Its oversight ensures that schools maintain high standards for curriculum, faculty, facilities, and clinical opportunities. Graduates from LCME-accredited schools are automatically eligible for U.S. residency programs.

ACGME – Accreditation Council for Graduate Medical Education

The ACGME accredits residency and fellowship programs. It sets rules regarding duty hours, competency milestones, and program requirements. IMGs must complete training in an ACGME-accredited program to obtain U.S. licensure and board certification.

ECFMG – Educational Commission for Foreign Medical Graduates

The ECFMG plays a central role for IMGs. It certifies that international graduates are ready for U.S. residency by requiring:

- Passing scores on USMLE Step 1 and Step 2 CK
- Verification of medical school credentials
- Graduation from a school listed in the World Directory of Medical Schools

Without ECFMG certification, IMGs cannot apply for U.S. residency. This process ensures that international training is equivalent to U.S. standards.

How IMGs Fit Into the U.S. Medical Ecosystem

Workforce Contribution

Nearly one-quarter of practicing physicians in the U.S. are IMGs. They are especially critical in:

- Primary care (internal medicine, family medicine, pediatrics)
- Underserved areas, such as rural regions and inner-city clinics
- High-demand specialties, including psychiatry and geriatrics

Bridging Gaps

IMGs bring valuable linguistic and cultural skills. A physician from Mexico may better serve Spanish-speaking patients in Texas, while a Nigerian physician may be more familiar with conditions affecting African immigrant populations.

Challenges for IMGs

Despite their importance, IMGs face:

- Residency competitiveness: Certain specialties are nearly inaccessible
- Visa restrictions: J-1 and H-1B visas limit flexibility
- Bias: Some program directors prefer U.S. graduates, assuming IMGs are less prepared

Strengths IMGs Bring

On the other hand, IMGs:

- Demonstrate resilience and adaptability
- Bring global perspectives on disease
- Provide essential services in communities underserved by U.S. graduates

Conclusion

Understanding the U.S. medical system is the first step for IMGs hoping to thrive. The journey is not just about exams and applications, it is about learning to operate in a system that prizes patient-centered care, team collaboration, and rigorous accreditation.

As an IMG, you may initially feel like an outsider. However, remember this: the U.S. healthcare system relies heavily on IMGs. Your background, skills, and determination are not weaknesses but assets. By understanding how the system works, its education pathways, healthcare delivery, accreditation bodies, and workforce dynamics, you will be better equipped to navigate it with confidence.

The road ahead will demand persistence. But just as you once learned anatomy, physiology, and clinical reasoning, you can learn the structures and culture of U.S. medicine. This chapter lays the foundation for everything that follows in this book: preparing before arrival, excelling in exams, securing clinical experience, and ultimately, finding your place in American medicine.

Chapter 2:
Preparing Before Arrival

Relocating to the United States to pursue medical training is one of the most important and life-shaping decisions an International Medical Graduate (IMG) can make. Before setting foot on American soil, a tremendous amount of preparation is necessary to ensure eligibility, competitiveness, and a smooth transition.

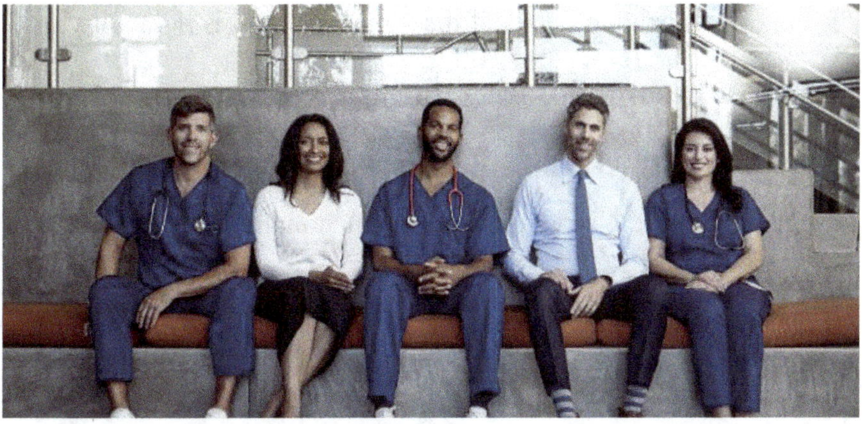

This chapter explores the essential steps and decisions IMGs must consider before arrival, from choosing the U.S. as a destination to credentialing, documentation, visas, and language proficiency.

Choosing the U.S. as Your Destination

For many international medical graduates, the United States stands out as the ultimate destination for medical training and practice. The reputation of American residency programs, the promise of cutting-edge facilities, and the potential for rewarding careers all make the U.S. an attractive choice.

Yet, the decision is rarely simple. It comes with significant challenges, financial, cultural, and personal, that deserve careful consideration.

Let us explore the pros and cons of choosing the U.S., followed by a comparison with other popular destinations such as the United Kingdom, Canada, and Australia. By weighing these factors, you'll be better equipped to decide if the American path is right for you.

Advantages of Choosing the U.S.

1. High-Quality Training

U.S. residency programs are internationally respected for their structured approach and emphasis on competency-based education. The Accreditation Council for Graduate Medical Education (ACGME) ensures that every program meets strict standards.

Residents are evaluated across multiple domains, such as medical knowledge, patient care, professionalism, communication, and systems-based practice. This structured training provides IMGs with a clear roadmap for their progression and skill development.

Compared to less standardized systems in other countries, the U.S. provides consistency across programs, which gives graduates confidence that they are meeting global standards.

2. Exposure to Cutting-Edge Technology and Research

Many of the world's leading hospitals and research centers are based in the U.S., including Mayo Clinic, Cleveland Clinic, Johns Hopkins, and Harvard-affiliated institutions. These centers are often at the forefront of clinical trials, advanced surgeries, and innovative treatments.

For IMGs, training in such environments provides exposure to:

- Robotic surgeries and minimally invasive techniques
- State-of-the-art imaging technologies
- Genomic medicine and personalized therapies
- Opportunities to participate in high-impact research publications

Such exposure doesn't just enhance technical skills; it also builds credibility for future international opportunities.

3. Strong Career Opportunities

A U.S. residency significantly enhances employability worldwide. Hospitals in the Middle East, Asia, and even Europe often view U.S.-trained physicians as highly competitive.

Moreover, many IMGs choose to remain in the U.S. after completing their training. For those who stay, opportunities range from academic medicine and research to private practice, offering diverse career trajectories.

4. Financial Rewards

While residency salaries in the U.S. (averaging $60,000 to $70,000 annually) are modest, the long-term earning potential is among the highest in the world.

Practicing physicians can earn:

- $200,000 to $300,000 annually in primary care
- $400,000 plus in surgical specialties and procedural fields

These figures are often two to three times higher than comparable positions in many countries. For IMGs supporting families or managing student debt, this is a major factor in choosing the U.S.

5. Diverse Patient Population

The U.S. is one of the most multicultural nations in the world. Physicians routinely care for patients from every ethnicity, religion, and socioeconomic background.

This diversity strengthens cultural competence, an essential skill for modern physicians. An IMG who trains in the U.S. will encounter:

- Language barriers requiring interpreters
- Health beliefs shaped by cultural traditions
- Socioeconomic challenges like lack of insurance or unstable housing

Learning to navigate these factors helps IMGs develop adaptability that serves them throughout their careers.

Challenges of Choosing the U.S.

While the advantages are compelling, the U.S. path comes with real difficulties. Understanding them upfront helps IMGs prepare mentally, financially, and emotionally.

1. Financial Costs

Applying for residency in the U.S. is expensive. Costs include:

- USMLE Step 1, Step 2 CK, and Step 3 exams (each $1,000+)
- ECFMG certification fees
- Travel and accommodation for interviews
- Visa application costs

Altogether, the total investment can exceed $15,000–$20,000 before residency even begins. For many IMGs, this is a major barrier.

2. Visa Restrictions

Many IMGs enter on J-1 or H-1B visas, which come with limitations.

- J-1 visas require physicians to return to their home country for two years after training unless they secure a waiver.
- H-1B visas depend on employer sponsorship, limiting flexibility.

Navigating immigration law often adds stress during training.

3. Highly Competitive Residency Match

Even though IMGs make up around 25% of the U.S. physician workforce, the match process remains fiercely competitive. Some specialties, like dermatology, orthopedic surgery, and plastic surgery, are almost inaccessible to IMGs.

Most IMGs find their best chances in primary care specialties (internal medicine, family medicine, pediatrics) or psychiatry. This reality means you may need to adjust career aspirations when entering the system.

4. Cultural and Social Adjustment

Adapting to life in the U.S. can be challenging. IMGs often face:

- Culture shock in day-to-day life
- Different expectations around communication and hierarchy in hospitals
- Feelings of isolation when far from family

These adjustments can be emotionally draining, especially during the intense years of residency.

5. Documentation and Exam Hurdles

Unlike many countries, the U.S. requires standardized licensing exams (USMLE series). Passing these exams requires not just medical knowledge but also test-taking strategies. Many IMGs must take time away from clinical practice to study full-time, which can be a difficult adjustment.

Choosing the U.S. as a destination for medical training offers world-class education, strong career prospects, and financial rewards. However, IMGs must also consider the financial, cultural, and bureaucratic challenges involved.

The U.S. is not the right choice for everyone. Some may find that the UK, Canada, or Australia offers a better balance of accessibility, lifestyle, and professional fulfillment.

Ultimately, the decision depends on your personal goals, resources, and resilience. If you are prepared for the challenges, the U.S. can provide unmatched opportunities that shape your career for decades to come.

Alternatives: UK, Canada, and Australia

United Kingdom

The UK attracts many IMGs because of the National Health Service (NHS), which offers a single nationalized employer. IMGs must typically pass the PLAB exam (Professional and Linguistic Assessments Board) and apply for training posts.

Pros include structured training, free healthcare access for residents, and easier immigration compared to the U.S.

However, competition is stiff, pay is lower than the U.S., and progression to consultant level can take longer.

Canada

Canada offers high-quality training, but IMG opportunities are limited due to restricted residency spots. Passing the Medical Council of Canada Qualifying Examination (MCCQE) is required.

While salaries are lower than the U.S., quality of life is often considered better, with universal healthcare and less medical litigation.

Australia

Australia is attractive for its relatively straightforward pathway for IMGs compared to North America. The AMC exams (Australian Medical Council) are required. Work-life balance is emphasized, but long-term residency and specialist training positions may be limited.

In short, choosing the U.S. offers world-class training and career benefits but comes with significant competition and financial investment. The decision must be carefully weighed against personal goals and circumstances.

Credential Evaluation: Laying the Groundwork

Before international medical graduates can even think about applying for residency in the United States, one critical step must be completed: credential evaluation and verification. This step establishes the validity, authenticity, and comparability of your medical education with U.S. standards. Without this foundation, your application cannot move forward.

Two major entities come into play: World Education Services (WES) and the Educational Commission for Foreign Medical Graduates

(ECFMG). While WES is often optional and used for broader educational or career purposes, ECFMG certification is mandatory for any IMG who wishes to enter residency training in the U.S.

This section unpacks what these organizations do, the requirements they enforce, the processes involved, and the strategies IMGs should use to avoid costly delays.

World Education Services (WES)

World Education Services is a nonprofit organization that specializes in evaluating academic credentials from outside the U.S. Its goal is to provide equivalency reports that translate international degrees and transcripts into U.S. educational terms.

For IMGs, WES is not required for medical licensure or residency applications. Instead, it is most relevant if you:

- Are applying for non-clinical graduate programs (e.g., Master of Public Health, Master of Business Administration).
- Want to pursue research fellowships or Ph.D. programs.
- Need academic equivalency reports for immigration, employment, or other professional purposes.

Many IMGs consider WES evaluations if they want to keep backup career pathways open outside clinical medicine, such as in healthcare management, policy, or education.

The WES process generally involves:

1. **Creating an account:** You register online and indicate the purpose of evaluation (education, immigration, or employment).
2. **Submitting transcripts and diplomas:** These must be sent directly from your medical school. WES does not accept photocopies sent by applicants.
3. **Evaluation report:** WES issues a document that outlines the U.S. equivalency of your medical degree. For example, an MBBS may be reported as equivalent to a U.S. Doctor of Medicine (MD).

Turnaround times range from 7 to 10 business days after receipt of all documents, though delays are common if schools are slow in responding.

When WES Is Useful for IMGs

While WES is not part of the ECFMG pathway, it can serve as a strategic tool. For example:

- If an IMG applies to an MPH program in the U.S. while preparing for USMLE exams, a WES evaluation is often required.
- Some research institutions request WES verification before offering positions to IMGs.

- Immigration-related processes, such as obtaining permanent residency through employment, sometimes require WES equivalency reports.

In short, WES should be seen as an adjunct, not a substitute, for ECFMG requirements.

ECFMG Certification Requirements

Unlike WES, ECFMG certification is non-negotiable for IMGs who want to enter U.S. residency programs. Established in 1956, ECFMG's mission is to ensure that foreign-trained physicians meet the same academic and professional standards as U.S. graduates.

Without an ECFMG certificate, you cannot apply for the National Resident Matching Program (NRMP), which is the official residency match system.

Medical School Recognition

The first requirement is that your medical school must be listed in the World Directory of Medical Schools (WDOMS) with an official ECFMG sponsor note.

- If your school is not listed or lacks a sponsor note, you are ineligible for certification, regardless of your personal achievements.
- This step ensures that only graduates of recognized, accredited medical institutions can pursue U.S. training.

Tip: Check WDOMS early, even before graduation, to confirm your school's status.

Primary Source Verification

ECFMG requires that your documents, diplomas, final-year transcripts, and proof of graduation, be sent directly from your medical school to confirm authenticity. This is called primary source verification.

- Photocopies or notarized documents are not accepted.
- The verification process can take several months, depending on how quickly your school responds.
- ECFMG communicates directly with your medical school through its secure systems.

Tip: Start this process as early as possible, preferably in your final year of medical school, since administrative delays are common.

Required Examinations

Examinations are the core of ECFMG certification. They ensure that IMGs demonstrate knowledge and clinical skills equivalent to U.S. medical graduates.

- **USMLE Step 1:** Tests basic sciences, such as anatomy, physiology, pharmacology, and pathology.
- **USMLE Step 2 Clinical Knowledge (CK):** Focuses on clinical sciences, diagnosis, and management.

- **USMLE Step 2 CS:** Formerly assessed clinical skills and patient interactions but was discontinued in 2021.
- **USMLE Step 3:** Required later for independent licensure but not for initial ECFMG certification.

Passing Step 1 and Step 2 CK is mandatory before you can obtain ECFMG certification.

EPIC System (Electronic Portfolio of International Credentials)

To modernize credential verification, ECFMG now uses the EPIC system.

- IMGs upload scanned copies of their credentials.
- ECFMG then contacts the issuing medical school to confirm the authenticity of the documents.
- Once verified, these documents remain stored digitally in your portfolio and can be shared with licensing boards and institutions.

This system reduces fraud and provides an accessible, long-term record of your credentials.

Common Pitfalls in Credential Evaluation

Even though the requirements are clear, many IMGs encounter challenges that delay or derail their applications. Some common pitfalls include:

1. Slow medical school administration: Some schools take months to respond to ECFMG requests.
2. Incomplete documentation: Missing seals, signatures, or incorrect formats often result in rejections.
3. Name discrepancies: Variations in the spelling of names on passports, diplomas, or transcripts can create verification issues.
4. Expired exam scores: USMLE scores remain valid for a limited period for ECFMG certification purposes.

Tip: Always double-check document requirements on the ECFMG website before submitting anything.

Strategic Considerations for IMGs

Credential evaluation is not just a bureaucratic step, as it can shape the trajectory of your U.S. medical career. Here are some strategic considerations to keep in mind:

- Start early: Begin credential verification well before residency application deadlines.
- Organize finances: Expect to spend thousands of dollars on fees for exams, verification, and certification.
- Backup plans: Use WES evaluations to explore academic alternatives in case residency is delayed.

- Networking: Connect with other IMGs from your school who have successfully completed the process; they often know how to expedite paperwork.

Case Example: Dr. Shao's Journey

Dr. Shao, an IMG from China, began preparing for U.S. residency during his final year of medical school. He checked WDOMS early to confirm his school's ECFMG eligibility. By the time he graduated, he had already submitted his transcripts to ECFMG through the EPIC system.

Despite his proactive approach, his school's administration delayed confirming his documents for nearly six months. This pushed back his USMLE Step 2 CK exam scheduling, almost making him miss the residency application cycle.

His experience highlights the importance of early action and persistence in credential evaluation.

This suggests that credential evaluation is the foundation of the U.S. residency journey. While WES offers flexibility for academic and career opportunities outside medicine, ECFMG certification is the non-negotiable gateway for clinical training.

The process may seem bureaucratic, but it serves a vital purpose: ensuring that all physicians entering the U.S. system meet the same rigorous standards as their American counterparts.

By starting early, preparing thoroughly, and anticipating delays, IMGs can navigate credential evaluation successfully and set themselves up for the next step: excelling in the U.S. residency match.

Gathering Transcripts, Diplomas, and Letters of Recommendation

For international medical graduates, preparing for the U.S. residency application process is as much about document management as it is about passing exams.

The transition from medical school abroad to a residency program in the United States requires that every credential, transcripts, diplomas, and letters of recommendation (LoRs), be carefully collected, authenticated, and presented in a format that U.S. institutions can recognize and trust.

Unfortunately, this step is often underestimated. Many applicants assume they can request transcripts or letters at the last moment, only to discover that bureaucratic delays, translation issues, and differences in academic culture can set their applications back by months, or even derail an entire application cycle.

This section provides a detailed roadmap for obtaining, organizing, and strategically using transcripts, diplomas, and recommendation letters in a way that strengthens your residency application.

Transcripts and Diplomas

Transcripts and diplomas serve as primary proof of your medical education. In the U.S. residency application process, these documents confirm:

- The legitimacy of your medical school and its recognition by ECFMG.
- Your academic progress, including courses, grades, and dates of attendance.
- That you have formally graduated and earned a medical degree equivalent to the U.S. MD or DO.

ECFMG requires these documents to undergo primary source verification, meaning they must come directly from your medical school and not through you. This requirement exists to prevent fraud and ensure uniform standards.

Common Challenges in Obtaining Transcripts

Administrative Delays

Some universities issue transcripts only once or twice a year. Also, smaller or rural institutions may lack dedicated offices for international credential requests.

In-Person Requests

In countries like India, Nigeria, or parts of the Middle East, schools often require the graduate to be physically present or to send an authorized family member with power of attorney to collect official transcripts.

Language Barriers

Transcripts in non-English languages must be translated by certified translation services, which adds time and cost.

Lost or Incomplete Records

In certain regions, older records may not be digitized, leading to missing grades or incomplete course lists.

Costs

Universities may charge processing fees. Add to this courier charges for international delivery, notarization fees, and translation services, and costs can easily run into several hundred dollars.

Best Practices for Obtaining Transcripts and Diplomas

- Start early: Begin the process at least 12 to 18 months before your residency application.
- Confirm ECFMG requirements: Ensure your school sends documents in the format and method required by ECFMG.
- Certified translations: Use only translators recognized by ECFMG; uncertified translations may be rejected.
- Keep personal copies: While ECFMG requires sealed envelopes sent directly, you should also keep certified copies for personal records.

- Track deliveries: Use couriers with tracking options to avoid lost documents.

Case Example:

Dr. Karim, an IMG from Egypt, requested his transcripts only four months before residency applications opened. His school delayed issuing them, and when the documents finally arrived, they were in Arabic. The certified translation took another eight weeks, causing him to miss that year's Electronic Residency Application Service (ERAS) deadline.

Letters of Recommendation (LoRs)

Unlike transcripts and diplomas, which serve as objective evidence of your education, letters of recommendation provide a subjective but powerful endorsement of your professional qualities, clinical competence, and personal character.

Residency program directors consistently rank LoRs among the top factors in evaluating applicants. Strong letters can make an average application stand out, while generic or weak letters can diminish even the most stellar USMLE scores.

Types of LoRs

U.S. Letters of Recommendation

- Most valuable in residency applications.
- Demonstrate that you have been evaluated by U.S. physicians who understand the expectations of American residency programs.

- Typically obtained during observerships, externships, sub-internships, or clerkships in the U.S.

Home Country Letters

- Provide useful context but usually carry less weight.
- More impactful if the recommender is an internationally recognized physician or if the letter demonstrates excellence in a specialty directly relevant to your application.

Hybrid Approach

- Many successful IMGs use a combination of U.S. and home country letters.
- Example: Two U.S. letters from observerships + one home country letter from a former professor who supervised original research.

What Makes a Strong LoR?

- Specificity: Generic statements like "hardworking and diligent" add little value. A strong letter cites concrete examples: a complex patient you managed, research you contributed to, or a leadership role you took.
- Context: The letter should explain the recommender's relationship to you (for example, "supervising physician during a 3-month internal medicine observership").
- Comparison: Strong letters place you in context (for example, "one of the top 5% of students I have mentored in 20 years").

- Understanding of U.S. standards: U.S.-based recommenders usually know how to frame their evaluations in terms residency directors value, teamwork, communication skills, adaptability to the U.S. system.

Securing Strong LoRs: Step-by-Step

1. Plan early: Identify opportunities for observerships or clerkships in the U.S. at least a year before applying.
2. Perform well: Treat every observership as an extended audition. Show professionalism, reliability, and initiative.
3. Ask directly and politely: When requesting a letter, approach mentors personally (in writing and verbally), providing them with your CV and personal statement to make their task easier.
4. Use ERAS LoR Portal: Letters must be uploaded directly by the recommender through ERAS, not handled by the applicant.
5. Diversify: If applying to internal medicine, for instance, secure at least two LoRs from internal medicine physicians and one from a related specialty (e.g., cardiology).

Tip: Avoid "committee-style" letters signed by multiple faculty. Residency directors generally prefer individualized evaluations.

Common Pitfalls with LoRs

- Asking too late, leaving recommenders rushed.
- Letters that are too short or vague.

- Using only home country letters.
- Not confirming whether the recommender actually submitted the letter.

Visa Categories and Their Implications

Visa choice is another make-or-break factor for IMGs. Even with stellar credentials, failure to secure the right visa can block access to residency programs. Understanding the differences between J-1, H-1B, and F-1 visas helps applicants align immigration pathways with career goals.

The J-1 visa (Exchange Visitor Visa) is the most common option for international medical graduates (IMGs) entering U.S. residency programs. It is sponsored by the Educational Commission for Foreign Medical Graduates (ECFMG) and comes with specific conditions. One of the most significant requirements is that physicians must return to their home country for two years after completing their training unless they are granted a waiver.

The J-1 visa offers several advantages. It is universally accepted by residency programs, making it the most straightforward pathway for many IMGs. The application process is simpler and faster compared to the H-1B visa, and the upfront costs are generally lower. However, the visa also has notable drawbacks. The two-year home residency rule can be restrictive, especially for those hoping to establish long-term careers in the United States. While waivers are available, they usually require physicians to work in underserved areas of the U.S. for about three years, which may not always align with personal or professional aspirations.

In contrast, the H-1B visa (Specialty Occupations) allows IMGs to complete residency without the obligation of returning home for two years. This visa, however, requires sponsorship from the residency program, and not all programs are willing or able to provide this support. Additionally, applicants are typically required to pass USMLE Step 3 before the H-1B can be issued.

The H-1B visa offers greater long-term career stability and makes the transition to permanent residency smoother compared to the J-1. On the downside, fewer residency programs sponsor this visa, and the application process involves more paperwork, higher legal fees, and greater administrative complexity.

The F-1 visa (Student Visa) is another pathway, though it is not directly applicable to residency training. Instead, it is typically used by IMGs who pursue further academic programs in the U.S., such as a Master of Public Health (MPH) or Ph.D., prior to residency applications. While it does not permit direct entry into residency, it can serve as a stepping stone for candidates seeking to strengthen their applications and build networks in the U.S. medical system.

When planning visa strategies, IMGs must weigh both short-term and long-term considerations. It is important to carefully research residency programs, as some explicitly state which visas they accept.

Those aiming for the H-1B should prioritize completing Step 3 early to remain eligible.

Finally, long-term goals should guide visa choices: while the J-1 may be the easier option for immediate residency entry, the H-1B often provides more stability for those hoping to establish their careers permanently in the United States.

Language Proficiency: TOEFL and IELTS

Although most IMGs study medicine in English, some states, programs, or visa categories require proof of English proficiency. Beyond exams, residency programs expect IMGs to communicate clearly with patients and colleagues.

The TOEFL (Test of English as a Foreign Language) is one of the most widely recognized exams for assessing English proficiency among international medical graduates (IMGs). It is accepted by the Educational Commission for Foreign Medical Graduates (ECFMG) and evaluates four key skills: reading, listening, speaking, and writing. The exam is available worldwide in an internet-based format, making it accessible for applicants across different regions.

Another option is the IELTS (International English Language Testing System), which some residency programs and institutions accept as an alternative to TOEFL. Like TOEFL, it measures proficiency across the same domains, reading, listening, speaking, and writing, but uses a slightly different scoring method.

Some candidates prefer IELTS depending on availability, cost, or familiarity with its format.

However, exams are only one part of the language challenge. Communication in residency extends far beyond test performance.

Even IMGs who are fluent in English often face difficulties adapting to the U.S. medical environment. One common challenge is medical jargon, as terminology can vary significantly between countries.

Another is patient interaction, where physicians must learn to explain complex conditions in simple, layman's terms that patients can easily understand.

Additionally, cultural nuance plays a big role. Residents must adapt to slang, idioms, and cultural references that shape how patients describe their symptoms or understand medical advice.

A useful strategy is to practice clinical English in real-life or simulated settings. Patient role-plays, clinical simulations, and shadowing opportunities help IMGs build confidence in bedside communication.

Ultimately, residency programs value not only strong exam scores but also a physician's ability to communicate with empathy, clarity, and cultural sensitivity.

Gathering transcripts, diplomas, and recommendation letters may seem bureaucratic, but it represents the foundation of an IMG's U.S.

residency application. Combine these with a clear visa strategy and strong language proficiency, and you will have a well-rounded application portfolio that reassures program directors of your readiness to train and practice in the United States.

Conclusion

Preparing to enter the U.S. medical system requires strategic planning years in advance. From carefully choosing the U.S. as the destination to securing ECFMG certification, gathering documents, planning for visas, and demonstrating language proficiency, IMGs must invest time, energy, and resources.

While the process is demanding, thorough preparation before arrival ensures smoother integration into the American system. For those who succeed, the rewards are substantial: access to world-class training, professional growth, and opportunities to serve diverse patient populations.

Chapter 3:
First Steps in the U.S.

Moving to the United States for residency is both an exciting and overwhelming milestone for international medical graduates (IMGs).

For many, it represents the culmination of years of hard work, passing licensing exams, preparing documents, and navigating visas. Yet the real transition begins after arrival, when academic preparation must translate into day-to-day adaptation.

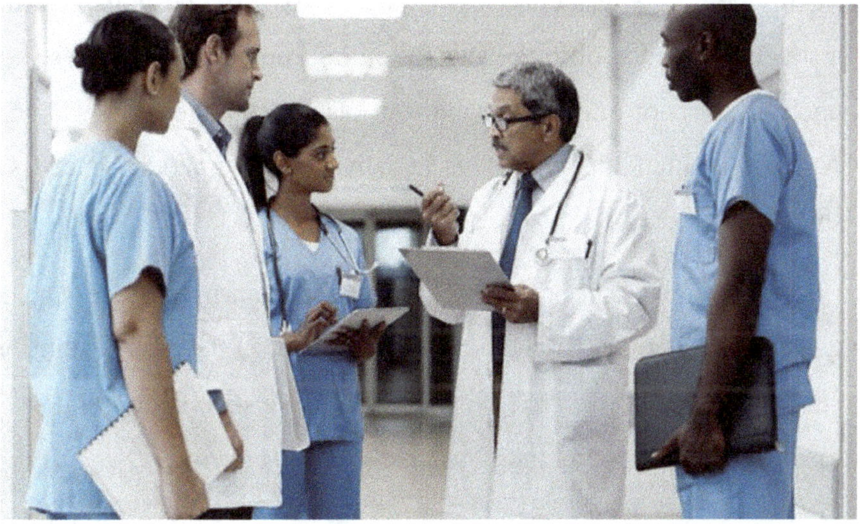

This chapter explores the early steps that IMGs must take in the U.S., from adjusting to cultural differences in medicine to practical necessities like housing and banking, to building social networks and coping with culture shock.

Adapting to Cultural Differences in Medicine Communication Styles

For many international medical graduates, one of the first hurdles after starting residency in the United States is learning how to navigate the different styles of communication within hospitals.

American medical culture places a strong emphasis on directness, clarity, and teamwork. This can be an adjustment for those who come from systems where deference to authority is the norm and where questioning a senior's instructions may be viewed as disrespectful.

In the U.S., residents are expected to ask questions, clarify instructions, and contribute actively during rounds. If an order seems unclear, it is not only acceptable but also encouraged to speak up. Attendings often appreciate this initiative because patient safety is a shared responsibility.

For example, a resident in China or Pakistan may be hesitant to question an attending's medication order, but in the U.S., failing to clarify a potentially unsafe dosage could have serious consequences for both the patient and the physician's training record.

Communication with patients also follows a different style. In many parts of the world, physicians are considered the unquestioned authority, and patients rarely challenge recommendations.

In contrast, American patients often want detailed explanations, alternative options, and opportunities to make informed choices. They may research conditions online before appointments and arrive with questions. While this can feel like a challenge to professional authority, it is a cultural expression of patient autonomy that U.S. doctors are trained to embrace.

Example: A patient with hypertension might ask, "What are the side effects of this drug? Are there natural alternatives? Could lifestyle changes be enough?" IMGs need to be ready to discuss these issues respectfully, even if, in their home country, such questioning would have been considered unusual or even inappropriate.

Hierarchy in U.S. Hospitals

Medical hierarchy exists everywhere, but the U.S. model is generally flatter and more collaborative than in many other countries. Attendings still hold ultimate responsibility, but residents, fellows, medical students, nurses, and physician assistants all play essential roles in patient care.

The expectation is that each member of the team will contribute their expertise.

Nurses, in particular, hold significant autonomy. In many states, nurse practitioners (NPs) and physician assistants (PAs) can prescribe medications, manage patients independently, and provide primary care. Even bedside nurses are empowered to question orders or escalate concerns about patient safety.

For IMGs accustomed to systems where nurses carry out physician orders without much input, this can feel surprising at first. However, collaboration with nursing staff is not optional. On the contrary, it is a critical part of the healthcare team's function.

Residents who build positive relationships with nurses and allied health professionals often find that their workdays run much more smoothly. Conversely, dismissing or undervaluing their input can damage a resident's reputation.

Understanding the dynamics of interprofessional collaboration early is essential for success.

Patient Interaction

Another important difference is the approach to patient interaction. In the U.S., the medical system is deeply invested in the concept of patient-centered care. Patients are encouraged to be active participants in their treatment decisions, and physicians are trained to facilitate shared decision-making.

A paternalistic style of medicine, common in parts of Asia, Africa, or the Middle East, where the doctor prescribes without discussion, is not well received in the U.S. Instead, IMGs must adopt communication strategies that reflect respect for autonomy: maintaining eye contact, using plain language instead of jargon, pausing to invite questions, and confirming that the patient understands the information before proceeding.

For example, if you recommend a surgical procedure, you must also explain the potential risks, alternatives, and what recovery may look like. Patients who feel excluded from decision-making are more likely to mistrust their physicians, seek second opinions, or even pursue legal action if something goes wrong.

This shift can be challenging for IMGs who trained in cultures where authority is rarely questioned. But with practice, many find that this approach builds stronger, more trusting patient relationships.

Cultural Competence

Perhaps the most profound adjustment for IMGs in the U.S. is treating patients from a wide range of ethnic, cultural, and linguistic backgrounds. Few countries are as diverse as the United States, where in a single clinic you might care for recent immigrants from Central America, refugees from the Middle East, long-time African American patients, and elderly White patients with rural backgrounds. Each group may carry unique cultural beliefs, expectations, and communication styles.

For instance, some families may prefer holistic or traditional remedies alongside prescribed medications. Others may have religious restrictions on treatments such as blood transfusions.

Some cultures may avoid discussing terminal illness directly, while U.S. medical ethics emphasize transparency about prognosis. Being sensitive to these differences does not mean compromising medical standards, but it does mean listening carefully, asking respectful questions, and incorporating patient preferences into the plan whenever possible.

A resident who adapts with empathy and flexibility not only improves patient rapport but also gains the respect of colleagues. Hospitals often provide cultural competence workshops, but much of the learning occurs at the bedside, through experience and reflection.

Navigating Life Outside the Hospital

Residency is not just about learning medicine. It also involves building a new life in a new country, often while under financial and emotional stress. For IMGs, everyday logistics can be as challenging as medical work. Managing these tasks early helps free mental space for residency duties.

Opening a Bank Account

One of the first steps upon arrival is opening a U.S. bank account. Without it, you cannot receive your residency salary or pay bills conveniently. Major banks such as Chase, Wells Fargo, and Bank of America often have programs tailored for newcomers, including international students and professionals.

To open an account, you will usually need your passport, visa, I-94 entry record, and proof of residence, such as a lease or utility bill. Some banks also ask for a Social Security Number (SSN). Since you may not have one immediately upon arrival, look for banks that allow account opening with just your passport and visa documents.

A practical tip is to compare fee structures before committing. Some banks charge monthly maintenance fees unless you maintain a minimum balance, while others waive fees for residents or students. Online-only banks and credit unions may offer better interest rates and lower fees, but large national banks have the advantage of wide ATM networks and customer service.

Housing

Finding housing is one of the more stressful tasks for new arrivals, especially in cities with high living costs such as New York, San Francisco, or Boston. Some hospitals provide subsidized housing or connect incoming residents with housing resources, but many IMGs must find rentals independently.

When choosing housing, consider proximity to the hospital, the safety of the neighborhood, access to public transportation, and overall affordability. Living close to the hospital may reduce commute stress, but it often comes at a higher rent. Sharing an apartment with other residents is a common strategy to keep costs manageable.

Connecting with current residents before arrival can be invaluable. They may know of available sublets, roommate opportunities, or neighborhoods that balance affordability with convenience.

Transportation

Transportation in the U.S. varies dramatically by region. In cities like New York, Chicago, or Boston, robust public transportation systems allow residents to live without a car. In smaller cities or suburban areas, however, owning a car is almost essential.

If you need to buy a car, budget not only for the purchase but also for insurance, which can be costly for newcomers without a U.S. driving history. Applying for a local driver's license soon after arrival can help reduce premiums. Be aware that each state has its own rules for converting foreign licenses, and some may require both written and road tests.

Social Security Number (SSN)

The Social Security Number is essential for almost every aspect of life in the U.S., employment, banking, taxes, credit, and sometimes even renting an apartment. Most residency programs guide new residents through the process, but it is your responsibility to apply soon after arrival. You will need your passport, visa documents, and I-94 entry record.

Without an SSN, you cannot be paid legally, so this step should be prioritized.

Credit History

In the U.S., credit history determines much more than eligibility for loans. Landlords, car insurance companies, and even some employers check credit scores. IMGs typically arrive with no U.S. credit record, which can make basic tasks like renting an apartment more difficult.

To start building credit:

- Apply for a secured credit card, which requires a deposit as collateral.
- Use it for small purchases and pay the balance in full every month.
- Pay all bills, such as utilities, rent, and phone, on time.

Within a year, you can begin to establish a strong credit history, which will make your financial life smoother in the long run.

Building a Support System

Residency in the United States is one of the most challenging periods in a physician's career.

The long hours, demanding workload, and constant learning curve are intense enough, but for international medical graduates, the challenges are multiplied by cultural transitions, adjusting to new systems, and the reality of living far from home.

In such a high-pressure environment, building a strong support system is not simply helpful, it is essential for both professional success and personal well-being.

Student and Resident Groups

One of the easiest entry points into building a community is joining student or resident organizations at the hospital or university where you train. Many institutions host international student and resident associations specifically to support IMGs. These groups can be a lifeline during your first months in the U.S.

Such associations often organize orientation sessions, provide guidance on housing and paperwork, and even host social activities like cultural dinners, hiking trips, or sports events. These interactions help break the ice, allowing IMGs to bond with peers facing similar challenges.

For example, new residents may feel overwhelmed by the sheer volume of administrative tasks like opening a bank account, applying for a Social Security Number, or setting up health insurance.

A well-established student or resident group often provides step-by-step guidance or even pairs new arrivals with a “buddy” who has gone through the same process. This mentorship dynamic helps flatten the learning curve and ensures newcomers do not feel lost in the bureaucracy.

IMG Networks

Beyond local hospital groups, IMG-focused professional networks play an important role in career growth and social integration.

The American Medical Association (AMA) IMG Section, for instance, organizes webinars, mentorship programs, and networking events specifically tailored to the needs of international doctors. Specialty-specific organizations, such as the American College of Physicians (ACP) or the American Academy of Pediatrics (AAP), often have dedicated spaces for IMGs, where members can exchange advice about board exams, career paths, and fellowship opportunities.

In the digital age, online communities are equally powerful. IMG WhatsApp groups, Facebook communities, and Reddit forums provide immediate answers to practical questions, anything from tips for preparing for USMLE Step 3 to where to buy affordable groceries near your hospital. Though informal, these networks are invaluable because they provide real-time peer support and an outlet for venting frustrations.

One advantage of these online communities is their diversity. A new resident in New York can share experiences with someone in California or Texas, gaining insights into different residency environments. This broad perspective helps IMGs anticipate challenges and discover solutions that may not be obvious within their own institution.

Alumni Associations

Another underutilized but highly effective resource is alumni associations. Many medical schools abroad have graduates who are now practicing in the U.S. and eager to help the next generation.

Alumni often understand the challenges of transitioning into American residency better than anyone else, since they once walked the same path.

These connections can open doors to research projects, observership opportunities, or career advice. For example, an IMG starting residency in internal medicine might reach out to an alumnus who is now a practicing hospitalist in the U.S. That alumnus may share insider knowledge on fellowship applications, strategies for networking at conferences, or pitfalls to avoid in the early years of practice.

In many cases, alumni mentorship extends beyond professional advice. They may also guide newcomers on housing options, navigating visa requirements, or finding cultural communities in a new city. The combination of career-focused and personal guidance makes alumni associations an invaluable part of a support network.

Family and Community

While professional groups provide mentorship and career support, family and community ties are critical for emotional stability. For IMGs who move with their spouse, children, or extended family, building a support system often involves finding schools, childcare, or local cultural communities that reflect their heritage.

For those arriving alone, connecting with cultural or religious communities, whether through local temples, mosques, churches, or cultural associations, can provide a sense of belonging. These groups often organize festivals, social gatherings, and community dinners that allow newcomers to experience a piece of home while forging new friendships.

Even simple routines, such as attending weekend community events or joining local hobby clubs (such as cooking classes, photography groups, or fitness groups), can significantly ease the transition. These social anchors reduce the sense of isolation that many IMGs experience and provide a healthier balance between work and personal life.

Overcoming Culture Shock and Isolation

Even with strong support systems, almost every IMG goes through some form of culture shock. Culture shock is not a sign of weakness. Rather, it is a natural response to adjusting to a new environment, culture, and lifestyle. The process often unfolds in predictable stages, and understanding these stages helps IMGs recognize that their struggles are normal and temporary.

Stages of Culture Shock

1. **Honeymoon Phase** – Upon arrival, everything feels exciting. The new environment, the advanced medical facilities, and the opportunities seem thrilling. This stage is filled with optimism and enthusiasm.

2. **Frustration Phase** – After the initial excitement, challenges set in. Language barriers, long work hours, unfamiliar systems, and separation from family begin to feel

overwhelming. This is often the hardest stage, marked by homesickness, irritability, or loneliness.

3. **Adjustment Phase** – Over time, routines are established, friendships form, and the new culture becomes more familiar. Frustrations decrease as coping strategies improve.

4. **Acceptance Phase** – Eventually, IMGs reach a stage of integration. They feel more confident navigating both residency and life in the U.S., blending aspects of their home culture with their new environment.

Common Challenges

- **Language barriers** – Even fluent English speakers may struggle with regional accents, fast-paced clinical conversations, or slang. Adapting to medical jargon unique to the U.S. (such as "code blue" or "workup") takes time.

- **Workload intensity** – Residency in the U.S. is notorious for long hours, night shifts, and high patient loads. For IMGs coming from systems with different structures, this can feel overwhelming.

- **Social norms** – Casual interactions with colleagues or patients may include humor, idioms, or cultural references that are confusing. Misunderstandings can sometimes cause embarrassment or feelings of exclusion.

- **Homesickness** – Missing family, familiar foods, and cultural traditions is one of the most universal struggles for IMGs.

Special occasions such as birthdays, holidays, or religious festivals can feel particularly lonely.

Coping Strategies

1. **Seek mentorship**: Senior IMGs who have already completed residency are one of the most valuable resources. They can share tips for managing workload, navigating hospital systems, and balancing personal life. Mentorship not only provides practical advice but also reassurance that challenges can be overcome.

2. **Practice self-care**: Residency is physically demanding, but neglecting self-care can quickly lead to burnout. Prioritizing adequate sleep, maintaining a balanced diet, and scheduling time for exercise, even short daily walks, can help maintain energy and emotional resilience. Mindfulness practices such as meditation or yoga are increasingly popular among residents for managing stress.

3. **Stay connected with home**: Thanks to technology, staying in touch with family and friends back home is easier than ever. Regular video calls, messaging, and even sharing daily updates can ease feelings of isolation. Some IMGs set up fixed weekly times to talk with loved ones, creating a routine that provides stability amid the chaos of residency.

4. **Embrace local culture**: Engaging with the local environment can speed up the adjustment process. Exploring

neighborhoods, attending cultural events, trying new cuisines, or participating in community activities fosters a sense of belonging. Rather than viewing differences as obstacles, IMGs who approach them with curiosity often find joy in discovering new traditions.

5. **Professional support**: If feelings of anxiety, depression, or burnout become overwhelming, seeking professional help is both normal and encouraged.

Mental Health Awareness for IMGs in Residency

Residency in the United States is one of the most rewarding yet challenging phases in a physician's career. As discussed earlier, for international medical graduates, the pressures are even greater, as they must simultaneously master their clinical duties, navigate cultural adaptation, manage immigration or visa-related stress, and cope with distance from family and familiar support systems. Amid these challenges, mental health often becomes a silent struggle.

While stigma around mental health persists in many cultures, awareness is slowly increasing within the medical community in the U.S. Hospitals, residency programs, and professional organizations are now recognizing physician well-being as a critical factor in training and patient care.

For IMGs, understanding mental health resources, recognizing early warning signs of burnout, and developing strategies for resilience are essential steps toward not only surviving residency but thriving in it.

Why Mental Health Awareness Matters

Residency demands long hours, intense patient care responsibilities, and the constant need to absorb vast amounts of medical knowledge. The average resident works 60 to 80 hours per week, often with overnight shifts that disrupt normal sleep patterns. For IMGs, these challenges are layered with additional stressors, some of which have already been discussed.

Let us have a quick recap of how these challenges can have an adverse impact on their mental health:

- **Cultural adjustment:** Learning new communication styles, adapting to workplace hierarchies, and managing unfamiliar expectations.
- **Visa and immigration stress:** Concerns about staying in the U.S., fulfilling visa requirements, or securing waivers.
- **Isolation:** Distance from family and friends, limited social networks, and homesickness.
- **Bias and stereotypes:** Facing doubts about competence simply because of foreign training.

Unchecked, these pressures can lead to burnout, depression, or anxiety. Mental health awareness matters because a physician's well-being is directly linked to patient safety, professional performance, and long-term career satisfaction.

Understanding Burnout

One of the most common mental health challenges among residents is burnout, defined by three main dimensions:

1. **Emotional exhaustion** – feeling drained, fatigued, or unable to face another day at work.
2. **Depersonalization** – developing a detached or cynical attitude toward patients, colleagues, or one's work.
3. **Reduced sense of accomplishment** – feeling ineffective, unmotivated, or questioning whether one is making a difference.

Burnout is not simply "being tired." It is a chronic condition that can escalate to serious mental health issues if left unaddressed. For IMGs, burnout may also manifest as self-doubt about their decision to move to the U.S. or as guilt about being far from family.

Early Warning Signs of Burnout

- Constant fatigue despite adequate sleep.
- Irritability with patients, staff, or peers.
- Decline in academic performance or clinical attentiveness.
- Loss of enthusiasm for medicine.
- Withdrawing from social interactions.

Recognizing these signs early allows residents to take corrective action before the situation worsens.

The Stigma Around Mental Health

In many cultures, mental health is rarely discussed openly. Some IMGs may come from countries where seeking psychiatric help is seen as a weakness or where counseling services are scarce. Within medicine itself, a culture of resilience and self-sacrifice often discourages residents from admitting vulnerabilities.

IMGs may fear that seeking help could harm their professional reputation, jeopardize their residency evaluations, or even affect visa status. This fear of stigma often leads to silence, with many suffering in isolation rather than seeking support.

The reality, however, is that U.S. hospitals increasingly encourage residents to use available resources. Confidentiality is strictly protected, and seeking support does not automatically reflect negatively on a physician's career. On the contrary, many program directors value residents who take proactive steps to maintain their well-being.

Resources Available to Residents

Most U.S. hospitals and residency programs now offer structured support systems for mental health:

Confidential counseling services: Many institutions provide access to licensed therapists or psychologists. Sessions are confidential and typically free or low-cost for residents.

Employee Assistance Programs (EAPs): EAPs offer counseling, stress management workshops, and referrals to community services. They often cover both personal and professional concerns, including family stress, financial issues, or legal advice.

Wellness committees and peer support groups: Many residency programs have wellness committees that organize group activities, provide mentorship, and create safe spaces for discussing stress. Peer support groups allow IMGs to connect with colleagues who share similar struggles.

Physician wellness programs: Some hospitals run formal wellness programs, including mindfulness training, resilience workshops, and stress-reduction techniques.

National hotlines and resources The Physician Support Line in the U.S. is staffed by volunteer psychiatrists who provide free, confidential help. Other resources, like the National Suicide Prevention Lifeline, are available 24/7.

Conclusion

For IMGs, the first steps in the U.S. are about more than survival; they are about laying the foundation for a successful career and fulfilling life. By adapting to new communication styles, managing practical aspects of daily living, building strong networks, and maintaining mental resilience, IMGs can thrive in both their professional and personal journeys.

While challenges are inevitable, each hurdle, whether understanding a cultural nuance, navigating the credit system, or overcoming homesickness, contributes to growth. The key is balance: investing energy not only in professional excellence but also in personal well-being.

Residency is the gateway to a long and meaningful career in medicine. With preparation, adaptability, and support, IMGs can turn the initial challenges into opportunities for transformation.

Chapter 4:
The USMLE Roadmap

For International Medical Graduates, the U.S. medical licensing exams, better known as the United States Medical Licensing Examination (USMLE), are more than just a hurdle. They are the foundation of the residency application, shaping how program directors view a candidate.

While strong letters of recommendation, clinical experience, and personal statements matter, USMLE scores often serve as the first filter in residency selection.

This chapter provides a comprehensive roadmap for IMGs navigating the USMLE journey: from understanding each step and building effective study strategies, to managing finances and learning from the stories of those who've succeeded, or stumbled, before you. By the end of this chapter, you should feel equipped with the knowledge to create your own personalized USMLE plan.

Overview of the USMLE

The USMLE is a three-step examination series designed to assess a physician's ability to apply knowledge, concepts, and principles essential for safe and effective patient care. It is co-sponsored by the Federation of State Medical Boards (FSMB) and the National Board of Medical Examiners (NBME).

USMLE Step 1

Focus: Tests basic science concepts, including anatomy, physiology, pharmacology, microbiology, pathology, and behavioral sciences. It also integrates clinical correlations.

Format: Computer-based, one-day exam with approximately 280 multiple-choice questions divided into seven 60-minute blocks. The exam pattern may change in the future.

Scoring: Since January 2022, Step 1 has been pass/fail. This was a major shift, aimed at reducing stress and overemphasis on Step 1 scores. However, residency programs still scrutinize attempts and the timeline of completion.

Role for IMGs: Passing Step 1 is required before applying for Step 2 CK and is often seen as a marker of foundational knowledge. Even though it's pass/fail, IMGs must aim to clear it on the first attempt, since multiple failures can significantly weaken applications.

USMLE Step 2 CK (Clinical Knowledge)

Focus: Clinical sciences, including internal medicine, surgery, pediatrics, psychiatry, and obstetrics/gynecology. Emphasis is placed on diagnosis, management, and prognosis.

Format: Approximately 318 multiple-choice questions across eight 60-minute blocks in a one-day session.

Scoring: Provides a three-digit score. In 2025, competitive specialties (dermatology, radiology, orthopedics) often expect 250+, while primary care programs (family medicine, pediatrics, internal medicine) may accept scores around 220–230. For IMGs, a higher Step 2 CK score is often critical, since Step 1 no longer provides numerical differentiation.

USMLE Step 2 CS (Clinical Skills) – Retired

Historically, Step 2 CS assessed clinical and communication skills with standardized patients. It was permanently discontinued in 2021, partly due to the COVID-19 pandemic and longstanding criticisms of cost and limited availability.

Alternatives for IMGs: The ECFMG's Pathways program now evaluates clinical and communication skills through alternatives like

OET (Occupational English Test) Medicine and documentation of training. IMGs should carefully check the ECFMG website for the most current pathway requirements before applying for residency.

USMLE Step 3

Focus: Assesses whether a candidate can apply medical knowledge and understanding of biomedical and clinical science essential for unsupervised medical practice.

Format: Two-day exam.

- **Day 1 (Foundations of Independent Practice):** Multiple-choice questions covering basic medical and scientific principles.
- **Day 2 (Advanced Clinical Medicine):** Multiple-choice questions and computer-based case simulations (CCS), where you manage virtual patients.

Scoring: Reports a three-digit score. Passing Step 3 is often required for obtaining an H-1B visa for residency and for advancing to independent practice or fellowship.

Study Strategies, Timelines, and Resources

Preparing for the USMLE is one of the most important steps in the journey of an International Medical Graduate. For many, the USMLE is not only an academic challenge but also a test of discipline, consistency, and adaptability.

Since IMGs often come from diverse medical education systems, having a clear, well-structured study plan is essential. This section outlines strategies that have consistently worked, realistic timelines for each exam, and a breakdown of the most reliable resources used by successful candidates.

Understanding the Landscape

Unlike some medical school exams where rote memorization may suffice, the USMLE demands both deep conceptual understanding and clinical application. The examiners are not just testing knowledge but also your ability to think like a U.S. physician, integrating basic sciences with clinical reasoning.

Therefore, preparation must be active, not passive. Reading alone is rarely enough; working through clinical vignettes, timed practice exams, and adaptive learning tools is essential.

Building a Realistic Timeline

Every IMG's starting point is different. Some are fresh graduates with recent exposure to medical school content, while others may have been practicing for years and need significant review. Nonetheless, there are general benchmarks that can guide your timeline.

Step 1 (Basic Sciences): Typical duration: 6 to 12 months of full-time preparation.

Key factors: If you've recently completed medical school, you may lean toward the shorter end of the spectrum. If you've been out of school for a while, 9 to 12 months is more realistic. Goal: Ensure mastery of physiology, microbiology, pharmacology, pathology, and behavioral sciences. Since Step 1 is now pass/fail, the focus is on passing on the first attempt rather than chasing a high score.

Step 2 CK (Clinical Knowledge): Typical duration: 4 to 8 months of preparation. Key factors: Your clinical exposure plays a huge role. If you've had rotations or clerkships in the U.S., you may adapt faster. If not, expect to need more time to familiarize yourself with the U.S. style of clinical decision-making. Goal: This is now the most important scored exam for IMGs. A high Step 2 CK score is a critical differentiator in residency applications, especially in competitive specialties.

Step 3 (Independent Practice Readiness): Typical duration: 2 to 4 months, often while in early residency or between observerships. Key factors: Many IMGs take Step 3 for visa eligibility (H-1B sponsorship requires passing Step 3). It's also seen as a sign of commitment and capability. Goal: Demonstrate the ability to manage patients independently.

Pro tip: Always plan your study timeline backward from the residency application deadlines (ERAS typically opens in September). For example, if you need Step 2 CK results ready for your application, ensure your exam is scheduled at least 2 to 3 months before submission to allow for score reporting.

Essential Study Resources

While countless prep materials exist, successful IMGs consistently rely on a core set of gold-standard resources. Trying to use too many can lead to stress and wasted time.

UWorld Question Bank

- Universally regarded as the single most important resource.
- Provides thousands of practice questions in the exact style of the USMLE.
- Explanations are detailed, with educational objectives that reinforce concepts beyond just the correct answer.
- Best used in tutor mode early to learn concepts, and timed mode later to simulate real exam conditions.
- For Step 2 CK, UWorld is almost indispensable at present.

First Aid for the USMLE Step 1

- Often referred to as the "Bible" of Step 1.
- Serves as a high-yield review book that consolidates the most important concepts.

- Works best when paired with UWorld, students annotate *First Aid* with explanations and notes from practice questions.

NBME Practice Exams

- Created by the same body that designs the USMLE, making them the most predictive self-assessment tools.
- Should be taken periodically (every 4 to 6 weeks) to benchmark progress.
- Scores can guide whether you're ready to sit for the real exam or need more preparation.

Pathoma and Sketchy

- Pathoma is excellent for pathology review, with Dr. Sattar's clear explanations and integrated visuals.
- Sketchy Medical uses creative storytelling and visuals to help memorize microbiology, pharmacology, and immunology. IMGs often find this particularly helpful for subjects with heavy memorization.

Online MedEd (for Step 2 CK)

- Focuses on clinical reasoning and management.
- Simplifies complex topics like cardiology or endocrinology into digestible frameworks.
- Often used alongside UWorld for a more structured foundation.

AMBOSS

- Provides an extensive library and integrated Qbank.
- Particularly useful for Step 2 CK and Step 3 as a supplement to UWorld.
- Has a "learning card" feature that's great for quick review.

Effective Study Strategies

Active Question-Based Learning: Instead of passively reading or memorizing, prioritize practice questions. This trains your brain to think in the USMLE format and prepares you for exam-day stamina.

Spaced Repetition and Daily Review: Apps like Anki (flashcards) help reinforce high-yield facts using spaced repetition, ensuring information sticks long term. Many IMGs adopt community-made USMLE decks as a starting point.

Simulated Exam Conditions: Time management is critical. Practice full-length exams under timed conditions to build endurance. Step 1 and Step 2 CK can last up to 8 to 9 hours, so conditioning yourself is essential.

Integrating Multiple Resources: Don't read *First Aid* in isolation. Instead, connect it with UWorld questions, Pathoma videos, or NBME practice scores. Integration reinforces retention.

Setting Benchmarks: Take an NBME exam early to establish a baseline. Use periodic assessments to track improvement. Only schedule your USMLE test date when your practice scores are within 5–10 points of your target range.

Avoiding Common Pitfalls

Resource overload: Many IMGs buy every prep book available. The result is scattered knowledge and burnout. Stick to two to three main resources.

Underestimating time: Some assume prior clinical experience means less preparation. However, the USMLE is highly standardized and requires specific test-taking skills.

Neglecting mental health: Long study hours without rest lead to burnout. Regular breaks, exercise, and social connection are part of effective studying.

Ignoring weak areas: It's tempting to focus on strengths, but success depends on shoring up weaknesses. Use UWorld and NBME results to identify gaps.

Sample 12-Month Timeline (for Step 1 and Step 2 CK)

Months 1 to 3: Foundation phase. Light reading of *First Aid*, Pathoma, or Online MedEd. Begin UWorld slowly in tutor mode.

Months 4 to 6: Active learning phase. Increase UWorld questions per day, review explanations thoroughly, and annotate *First Aid*. Take the first NBME to gauge readiness.

Months 7 to 9: Intensify focus. Transition to timed blocks, simulate full-length exams, and address weak areas aggressively. Take additional NBME exams.

Months 10 to 12: Final review. Re-do incorrect UWorld questions, focus on Anki flashcards, and simulate full-length exams every 2 to 3 weeks.

This plan can be shortened or lengthened depending on your background, but the principle of cycles, foundation, active learning, and final review, should preferably remain the same.

Success on the USMLE requires more than intelligence. It requires a well-planned strategy. For IMGs, the exams are not just about testing medical knowledge but also about adapting to the expectations of the U.S. medical system. By sticking to core resources like UWorld, *First Aid*, and NBME exams, setting a realistic timeline, and committing to active learning, you can maximize your chances of success.

Remember: the exam journey is a marathon, not a sprint. Small, consistent progress each day compounds into mastery. Most importantly, don't compare your timeline with others. Your path is unique, and the right strategy for you is the one that balances preparation with well-being.

Common Challenges for IMGs in Preparation

For many international medical graduates, preparing for the USMLE is one of the most demanding experiences of their professional lives. The exams are not only academically rigorous but also embedded within a healthcare, educational, and cultural framework that may differ dramatically from what IMGs are accustomed to in their home countries.

Understanding these challenges upfront is crucial. Awareness helps reduce unnecessary stress, allows IMGs to plan better, and increases the likelihood of success.

1. **Academic and Knowledge Gaps:** Perhaps the most obvious challenge is the difference in medical curricula. Medical schools around the world vary widely in what they emphasize. While some focus heavily on basic sciences in the first few years and clinical medicine later, others integrate both throughout the program. The USMLE exams, particularly Step 1 and Step 2 CK, test knowledge in a very specific way, emphasizing clinical reasoning, integration of pathophysiology with patient management, and evidence-based medicine.

Many IMGs find that topics like biostatistics, epidemiology, ethics, and patient safety are underrepresented in their home curriculum. U.S. students are exposed to these subjects early, often alongside training in standardized test-taking strategies. For IMGs, catching up requires dedicated self-study and, often, learning from scratch.

2. **Adapting to Multiple-Choice Test Formats:** In many countries, medical school assessments are oral exams, essay-style tests, or practical clinical demonstrations. The USMLE, on the other hand, is entirely multiple-choice, with complex, scenario-based questions. These items often include long

vignettes with extraneous information, designed to mimic real-life patient encounters.

IMGs frequently underestimate the skill required to parse these questions effectively. Success depends not only on knowing the material but also on applying deductive reasoning quickly under time pressure. Without prior experience, IMGs may initially perform poorly even if they have strong medical knowledge. Developing this skill requires consistent practice through resources like UWorld and NBME practice exams.

3. **Language and Communication Barriers:** Even fluent English speakers may find USMLE preparation daunting. Medical terminology may be familiar, but test questions often include colloquial phrases, idiomatic expressions, or cultural references. For example, a patient may describe “heartburn after eating spicy wings” rather than “gastroesophageal reflux symptoms.” Recognizing these subtleties takes time.

Language barriers extend beyond the exams themselves. When preparing for clinical observerships or residency interviews, IMGs may struggle with conversational speed, regional accents, or humor. Misunderstanding a question during the exam or interview could negatively impact performance.

4. **Limited Access to High-Quality Resources:** U.S. medical students typically have institutional access to UWorld subscriptions, NBME practice tests, and review materials like *First Aid for the USMLE*. IMGs, especially those from low- or middle-income countries, often lack such institutional

support. These resources are expensive, and paying in U.S. dollars can be prohibitive.

Some IMGs resort to outdated or pirated materials, which may not reflect the current exam blueprint. This can create knowledge gaps or misaligned preparation. Financial constraints also limit the ability to attend live review courses, participate in question banks for extended periods, or travel to test centers.

5. **Financial Stress:** Finances represent one of the most significant challenges. Preparing for the USMLE is not just about purchasing study materials. It also includes exam registration fees, travel expenses, housing near test centers, and potentially giving up income during preparation.

As of 2025, the cost of each USMLE exam runs into hundreds of dollars, with Step 1 and Step 2 CK registration for IMGs each exceeding $1,000. Step 3 adds additional costs, not to mention the application fees for residency programs through ERAS. For IMGs who come from countries with weaker currencies, these expenses can equal several months, or even years, of savings.

Financial pressure compounds stress, sometimes forcing IMGs to juggle part-time work alongside exam preparation. This can prolong timelines and reduce study efficiency.

6. **Lack of Structured Guidance:** U.S. medical students prepare for the USMLE under structured curricula, with faculty advisors, academic coaches, and peer study groups. IMGs often prepare in isolation. Without mentors who

understand the system, IMGs may waste months using ineffective strategies or prioritizing low-yield topics.

The absence of clear, step-by-step guidance leads to uncertainty: How many NBME exams should I take? What is a competitive score for my specialty? How long should I study before attempting Step 1? The trial-and-error approach prolongs preparation and adds emotional strain.

7. **Visa and Immigration Concerns:** While not directly tied to studying, immigration issues weigh heavily on IMGs. Preparing for exams while simultaneously worrying about visa status, eligibility for observerships, or restrictions on travel creates an extra layer of stress. Some IMGs must leave their home country to sit for the exams, requiring careful planning and financial support.

The uncertainty of whether they will secure a visa for residency interviews can also impact motivation. Unlike U.S. graduates, IMGs face bureaucratic hurdles that extend beyond academics.

8. **Psychological and Emotional Stress:** The USMLE preparation process is mentally taxing for everyone, but IMGs face unique emotional challenges. Feelings of isolation are common, especially if studying away from family or in a new country. The fear of failure is magnified by the financial investment and the weight of representing one's family or community.

Burnout is a real risk. Long study hours, lack of social support, and high stakes contribute to anxiety and depression. IMGs may be reluctant to seek mental health support due to stigma or unfamiliarity with services in the U.S. This emotional burden can undermine focus and productivity.

9. **Balancing Work, Study, and Family:** Many IMGs cannot afford to dedicate themselves full-time to studying. They may need to work clinically in their home country, take on non-clinical jobs, or support family members financially. Balancing these obligations with intensive exam preparation is daunting.

IMGs with families face additional challenges. Parents may struggle to find quiet study time while caring for children. Spouses may feel neglected, leading to relationship strain. Without careful time management, personal responsibilities can derail even the most disciplined study plans.

10. **Variability in Preparation Timelines:** Unlike U.S. students who typically take Step 1 and Step 2 CK during medical school, IMGs may attempt these exams years after graduation. Medical knowledge fades over time, and revisiting basic sciences can feel like starting over.

Older graduates may also face implicit bias in residency applications, making high USMLE scores even more critical. This amplifies the pressure to perform, yet the longer gap since medical school makes preparation harder.

11. **Residency Application Pressure:** While the USMLE exams themselves are a hurdle, IMGs know that strong scores are just one piece of the puzzle. U.S. residency programs remain highly competitive, with preference often given to American graduates.

This knowledge fuels perfectionism. IMGs may feel that anything short of stellar scores will ruin their chances, creating a cycle of anxiety that affects exam performance. The high-stakes nature of the process can make it difficult to study with confidence.

12. **Navigating Online Communities and Information Overload:** In the absence of institutional support, IMGs often turn to online forums, YouTube channels, or WhatsApp groups for advice.

While these communities can be helpful, they can also spread misinformation. Conflicting opinions about which resources to use, how long to study, or what scores are competitive often leave IMGs confused.

Information overload leads to "resource hopping," where candidates abandon one strategy prematurely to try another. This inconsistency prevents mastery of key materials and wastes valuable time.

Preparing for the USMLE as an IMG is more than an academic challenge. It is a holistic struggle involving finances, culture, language, and mental health. Yet acknowledging these challenges is the first step toward overcoming them. With proper planning, mentorship, and resilience, thousands of IMGs successfully navigate this journey each year.

The key is to remember that challenges are not signs of inadequacy, they are shared experiences. By anticipating them, developing coping strategies, and seeking support, IMGs can transform obstacles into stepping stones toward their ultimate goal: practicing medicine in the United States.

Balancing Finances, Work, and Study

For international medical graduates, preparing for the U.S. medical licensing process is not only academically challenging but also financially demanding. Exam registration, study resources, travel, observerships, and application fees quickly add up.

Unlike U.S. medical students who may have access to loans or institutional support, IMGs often fund their journey independently, sometimes while working or supporting families. Balancing finances, work obligations, and intense study schedules becomes one of the greatest hurdles. This section explores the realities of that balance and strategies to make it more manageable.

1. **Understanding the Financial Burden:** The costs of the U.S. medical licensing journey can be significant. As of 2025, IMGs typically have to pay:

- USMLE Step 1 and Step 2 CK registration: $1,015 each.
- Step 3: $925.

- International test delivery surcharge: $200 to $300 per exam if taken outside the U.S. or Canada.
- Residency application fees (ERAS): $99 for the first 10 programs, then escalating fees for additional applications. Competitive specialties often require applying to 80 to 100 programs, pushing application costs into the thousands.
- NRMP Match registration: $70 to $150 depending on deadlines.
- Travel for observerships, electives, and interviews: often several thousand dollars.

When combined with resource subscriptions (UWorld, NBME exams, *First Aid* books, question banks), the total cost for an IMG from first exam to residency application can range from $15,000 to $25,000. For those coming from low- and middle-income countries, this represents several years' worth of savings.

2. **The Dilemma: Work vs. Study:** IMGs often face a difficult trade-off. On the one hand, full-time preparation may yield higher exam scores, but it eliminates the possibility of income. On the other hand, working while preparing provides financial stability but stretches timelines and increases fatigue.

Some IMGs continue working as doctors in their home countries, saving money while studying during evenings and weekends. Others take non-clinical jobs, such as research assistants, tutors, or unrelated work, to sustain themselves while abroad. Each option has advantages and drawbacks.

3. **Budgeting for the USMLE Journey:** Budgeting is one of the most powerful tools IMGs can use to stay on track. Creating a financial plan before starting prevents surprises and reduces anxiety.

4. **Affordable Resource Strategies:** IMGs often feel pressured to purchase expensive prep courses or multiple question banks. In reality, success comes from depth rather than breadth.

5. **Time Management While Working and Studying:** Balancing work and study requires careful scheduling. IMGs who succeed often treat preparation like a second job.

6. **Family and Social Pressures:** Many IMGs face pressure to provide financial support to family members while also investing in their own future.

7. **The Psychological Weight of Financial Stress:** Money worries do more than limit resources, they affect concentration and mental health.

8. **Leveraging Financial Support Options:** Though IMGs cannot access federal student loans in the U.S., several alternative funding sources exist.

IMGs who acknowledge challenges and prepare for them systematically are far more likely to succeed. The process is demanding, but it is also an investment. Each dollar, hour, and sacrifice contributes to the ultimate goal: earning the privilege to practice medicine in the United States.

Success Stories and Cautionary Tales

The journey from being a medical graduate abroad to becoming a practicing physician in the United States is full of challenges.

For some, careful planning, persistence, and a strong support network result in remarkable success. For others, missteps and lack of preparation serve as sobering lessons.

Examining real-world patterns and composite examples of international medical graduates helps highlight strategies that work, and pitfalls to avoid.

The Power of Persistence: A Success Story: Consider the case of Dr. Meera, a physician from India who dreamed of practicing internal medicine in the U.S. She graduated in 2016 and began her USMLE journey while working at a hospital in her hometown. Instead of rushing, she created a three-year plan: dedicate one year to Step 1, one year to Step 2 CK and electives, and the final year for Step 3 and applications.

Meera used trusted resources, UWorld, *First Aid*, and NBME self-assessments, and avoided the temptation to buy multiple question banks. She studied consistently, three hours each weekday and full days on weekends. She saved money by sharing resources with peers and budgeting for exam fees months in advance.

When applying for residency, she submitted to 120 internal medicine programs, including community hospitals and mid-tier academic centers. She tailored every personal statement, attended virtual open houses, and followed up with thank-you emails after interviews.

Her persistence paid off: Meera matched into her top-choice program in New Jersey. Today, she mentors other IMGs, emphasizing that success is less about brilliance and more about sustained effort, resilience, and organization.

Strategic Networking: A Success Story: Dr. Khafre, an IMG from Egypt, highlights the role of networking. After completing medical school, Khafre struggled to find research or observership opportunities in the U.S.

He started by joining the American College of Physicians (ACP) as a student member. Through ACP's IMG section, he attended webinars, connected with alumni from his medical school, and eventually secured a research position at a U.S. university hospital.

Though the stipend was modest, the experience gave him access to mentors, U.S. clinical experience, and letters of recommendation. Khafre balanced his work by waking at 5 a.m. daily to practice UWorld questions. He scored 245 on Step 2 CK and matched into an internal medicine residency at the same hospital where he had done research.

His story shows how strategic networking, not just high scores, can tip the scales in a competitive process. For IMGs, who often lack local connections, professional organizations and alumni associations can serve as crucial bridges.

A Cautionary Tale: Delayed Decisions: Not every IMG succeeds on the first attempt. Dr. Samantha, from Brazil, graduated in 2012 but postponed her USMLE exams repeatedly, waiting until she felt “perfectly ready.” She bought multiple prep courses but never completed them, rescheduling her exam dates each time. By 2018, she had not yet taken Step 1, and her year-of-graduation gap raised red flags with residency programs.

When she finally attempted Step 2 CK, her preparation was rushed. She failed by a small margin, losing exam fees and confidence. Though she eventually passed, by the time she applied for residency, her profile was considered “older,” and despite applying to 150 programs, she went unmatched twice.

Samantha’s case illustrates the dangers of perfectionism and procrastination. For IMGs, long graduation gaps reduce competitiveness. Residency directors often prefer recent graduates, and delays can close doors. The lesson: commit to a realistic timeline and stick to it.

Conclusion

The journey through the USMLE exams is far more than a series of tests. It is a transformative process that shapes the knowledge, resilience, and determination of international medical graduates.

From understanding the structure of Step 1, Step 2 CK, and Step 3, to navigating the complexities of study strategies, financial pressures, and cultural adjustments, this chapter has laid out both the roadmap and the realities of preparation.

For IMGs, the challenges can feel overwhelming: balancing work, limited finances, and personal obligations while striving to master the dense content of the exams. Yet, as the success stories show, perseverance, strategic planning, and adaptability can make the seemingly impossible attainable. On the other hand, the cautionary tales remind us of the importance of discipline, realistic timelines, and informed decision-making.

Ultimately, the USMLE process is not just about passing exams but about proving readiness to thrive in the U.S. healthcare system. Each step, whether challenging or rewarding, brings IMGs closer to their goal of practicing medicine in the United States. With the right resources, mindset, and support, the USMLE can serve as a stepping stone toward a fulfilling career that impacts countless patients' lives.

Chapter 5:
Clinical Experience in the U.S.

For international medical graduates, clinical experience in the United States is one of the most decisive factors in securing a residency position.

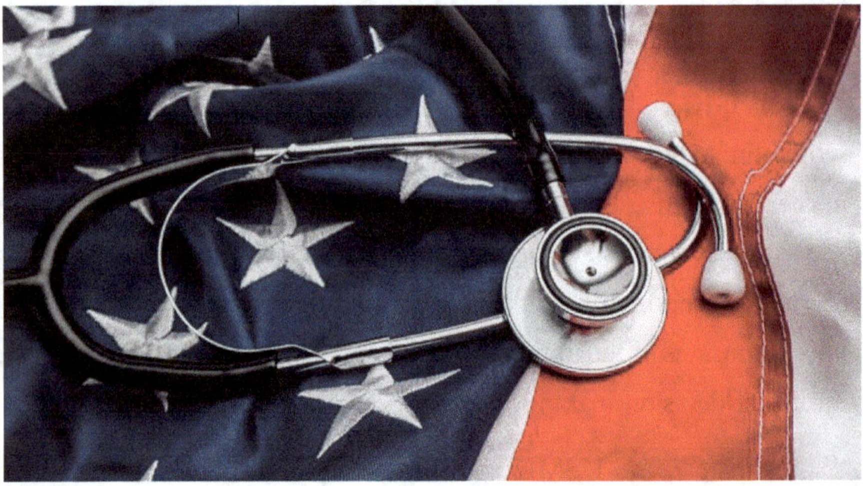

While excellent USMLE scores and strong academic records are important, program directors consistently emphasize that firsthand U.S. clinical training sets candidates apart. It not only demonstrates familiarity with the American healthcare system but also reassures programs that applicants can adapt to the cultural, ethical, and professional expectations of U.S. medicine.

This chapter explores the many dimensions of U.S. clinical experience and why it matters so profoundly for IMGs. We will begin by looking at the types of opportunities available, observerships, externships, clerkships, electives, and research fellowships, each offering different levels of exposure and responsibility. From there, we'll cover the practical steps of applying and securing placements, including strategies to make applications competitive and pitfalls to avoid.

Equally important is what happens during these experiences: networking with attendings and preceptors, building professional relationships, and earning strong documentation and letters of recommendation (LORs) that carry significant weight in residency applications.

By the end of this chapter, you will have a clear, step-by-step roadmap for turning U.S. clinical experience into one of the strongest assets of your journey from abroad to MD.

Why U.S. Clinical Experience Is Critical

For international medical graduates, the path to practicing in the United States does not only run through the United States Medical Licensing Examination (USMLE). Equally important is the acquisition of meaningful U.S. clinical experience (USCE).

Residency program directors consistently rank U.S. clinical experience as one of the most important criteria in evaluating IMG applicants. According to the National Resident Matching Program (NRMP) Program Director Survey (2022), over 80% of residency program directors cited clinical experience in the U.S. as an important factor in deciding whom to interview.

Why is this the case? The answer lies in how residency programs evaluate readiness. Medicine is not practiced in isolation, it is influenced by healthcare systems, cultural expectations, electronic medical record (EMR) use, and interdisciplinary teamwork. Even the language of medicine varies across borders.

For instance, while an IMG may be well-versed in pathophysiology and patient care in their home country, adapting to the American system requires a different set of competencies.

Some of the core reasons USCE is critical include:

Familiarity with the U.S. healthcare system: IMGs must learn how U.S. hospitals function, including EMRs like Epic and Cerner, HIPAA regulations, insurance-driven care models, and interprofessional dynamics.

Cultural competency: Patient interactions in the U.S. demand fluency not only in English but in nuances of patient-centered communication, shared decision-making, and documentation standards.

Letters of recommendation (LORs): U.S.-based LORs are often required by residency programs. Letters from preceptors or attendings who know the U.S. system carry much more weight than foreign recommendations.

Demonstrated commitment: Clinical experience in the U.S. signals to programs that the IMG is serious about practicing medicine here and has invested the time and effort to integrate into the system.

Residency interview performance: Firsthand experience provides IMGs with stories and examples to discuss during interviews. Talking about a U.S. patient encounter demonstrates readiness far better than citing only overseas experience.

In essence, U.S. clinical experience bridges the gap between theoretical preparation and real-world application. Without it, even a highly qualified IMG risks being overlooked during the residency match process.

Types of U.S. Clinical Experience

Not all clinical experiences are created equal. IMGs have multiple options, each with its own structure, benefits, and limitations. Understanding these distinctions helps applicants choose the best path for their circumstances.

Observerships

Definition: Shadowing physicians in clinical settings without direct patient care responsibilities.

Who qualifies: Typically open to IMGs who have graduated from medical school.

Pros: Provides exposure to U.S. healthcare, EMRs, and physician–patient interactions; often easier to secure than externships or clerkships.

Cons: Limited hands-on involvement; cannot perform physical exams or write notes.

Observerships are best for graduates seeking to demonstrate continued clinical engagement, especially if they have been out of practice. However, because they lack active involvement, residency directors may view them as less robust than other forms of USCE.

Externships

Definition: Structured programs that allow IMGs to participate in direct patient care, such as taking histories, performing physical exams, and documenting in EMRs (under supervision).

Who qualifies: Usually open to graduates rather than students.

Pros: Stronger letters of recommendation; hands-on experience mirrors residency responsibilities.

Cons: Can be competitive and costly; some require malpractice insurance coverage.

Externships are highly valuable because they demonstrate clinical competency in a U.S. setting. Many IMG-friendly programs value externship experience almost as highly as U.S. medical student clerkships.

Clerkships

Definition: Core or elective rotations undertaken by medical students, typically in their third or fourth year.

Who qualifies: Reserved for current medical students (including international students at recognized institutions).

Pros: Hands-on, integrated experience alongside U.S. medical students; ideal for building strong LORs.

Cons: Not available to graduates; limited to students from schools that have affiliation agreements with U.S. hospitals.

For IMGs still in medical school, arranging clerkships in the U.S. is one of the best strategies to secure meaningful USCE early.

Electives

Definition: Optional rotations chosen by students in specific specialties, usually during the final year of medical school.

Who qualifies: International medical students in their clinical years.

Pros: Opportunity to explore specialties, gain mentorship, and secure LORs tailored to residency applications.

Cons: Competitive; often require strong academic standing and proof of English proficiency.

Electives are especially helpful for IMGs targeting competitive specialties like dermatology, radiology, or cardiology.

Research Fellowships

Definition: Structured academic roles that involve clinical or laboratory research, often at academic medical centers.

Who qualifies: Open to both graduates and students.

Pros: Provides U.S.-based publications and networking opportunities; strengthens applications for research-heavy specialties.

Cons: May not count as clinical experience if no patient interaction is involved; often requires a significant time commitment.

While not a substitute for direct USCE, research fellowships are particularly beneficial for IMGs who aspire to academic careers or specialties with strong research components.

Networking with Attendings and Preceptors

For international medical graduates, clinical rotations are not only about learning the U.S. healthcare system but also about building relationships. Networking with attendings, fellows, residents, and even other international colleagues is one of the most powerful ways to strengthen your path toward residency.

In fact, surveys from the National Resident Matching Program (NRMP) consistently show that letters of recommendation and U.S. clinical evaluations rank among the top factors in residency selection. These only come when you connect meaningfully with mentors.

So how do you turn a short observership or externship into lasting professional connections? Let's walk through the strategies.

1. Why networking matters for IMGs

Networking in the U.S. medical environment is not about handing out business cards or adding people on LinkedIn. It's about earning trust and demonstrating your professionalism. When an attending or preceptor feels they can vouch for your clinical judgment, teamwork, and reliability, they are more likely to write you a strong letter of recommendation, introduce you to residency program directors, or even open doors to research collaborations.

Networking also helps IMGs:

- Learn unwritten rules of U.S. medical culture (communication style, hierarchy, expectations).
- Gain insight into residency programs, interviews, and specialty competitiveness.
- Build a support system for advice and encouragement throughout the stressful Match journey.

2. Professionalism: the foundation of all networking

Your reputation starts the moment you enter the hospital or clinic. Attendings and residents will notice not just your knowledge, but also your punctuality, attitude, and respect for team dynamics. Basic professionalism includes:

- Arriving on time (ideally 10 to 15 minutes early).
- Dressing appropriately (business casual or scrubs if required).
- Addressing staff formally ("Dr. Smith," "Dr. Rodriguez") unless invited to use first names.

- Being mindful of cultural differences in communication, U.S. medicine values conciseness, clarity, and patient-centered language.

Consistency in these small details builds trust and sets the tone for stronger networking opportunities.

3. Active engagement during rotations

Networking is strongest when you contribute value to the team. Even as an observer or extern, you can:

- Ask thoughtful questions, not just "What medication is that?" but "Why was this therapy chosen instead of the alternative?"
- Offer to help with tasks within your scope, summarizing charts, looking up guidelines, and preparing literature reviews.
- Show curiosity, attend grand rounds, morbidity and mortality conferences, or journal clubs, even if not mandatory.
- Take initiative, ask if you can present a short case or prepare a five-minute teaching point.

These actions demonstrate interest and seriousness, which preceptors remember.

4. Building rapport with attendings

Attendings are often busy, but most enjoy teaching motivated students. Practical tips for approaching them:

- Introduce yourself early: "Dr. Johnson, I'm Dr. Patel, an IMG from India here for an observership in cardiology. I'm very excited to learn from your team."
- Express specific interest: "I'm particularly interested in heart failure management, and I was hoping to observe how the team handles advanced therapies."
- Respect their time: keep questions concise and well-prepared; avoid catching them during high-stress patient care unless appropriate.
- Follow up on discussions: if an attending mentions a study, read it and bring it up later. This shows initiative.

5. Connecting with residents and fellows

Residents and fellows are often more accessible than attendings and can be invaluable mentors. They were recently in your shoes and understand the Match process well.

- Show interest in their career paths and ask for advice.
- Offer to help with research projects or case reports. Many publications start this way.

- Ask them for honest feedback on your performance and how to improve.

A strong resident advocate can sometimes influence attendings to write stronger letters on your behalf.

6. Networking beyond the hospital

Expand connections outside of direct rotations:

- **Academic events:** Attend grand rounds, CME events, or specialty society meetings. Even virtual webinars are useful.
- **Professional organizations:** Join groups like the American Medical Association (AMA), American College of Physicians (ACP), or specialty societies. Many offer discounted IMG memberships.
- **Online platforms:** LinkedIn and ResearchGate can help you stay connected with mentors after your rotation ends. Share updates respectfully, not excessively.

7. Following up and staying connected

Networking doesn't end when the rotation ends. Stay in touch in a professional, non-intrusive way:

- Send a thank-you email after your rotation, highlighting what you learned.
- Share periodic updates on milestones (passing USMLE exams, submitting applications, research accepted).

- Congratulate mentors on achievements (new positions, publications) via LinkedIn or email.

These small touches keep you on their radar without being overbearing.

Common Mistakes to Avoid

Networking can backfire if done poorly. Avoid:

- Asking for a letter of recommendation on your first day. Build rapport first.
- Overstepping boundaries (performing tasks not permitted).
- Over-communicating (daily emails or messages can be seen as unprofessional).
- Speaking negatively about other IMGs, hospitals, or programs.

Turning Networks into Opportunities

Effective networking leads to:

- Stronger, more personalized LORs.
- Invitations to research or case reports.
- Introductions to residency program directors.
- Long-term mentorship relationships.

Many IMGs who successfully match report that a mentor they met during a U.S. rotation was pivotal, either by writing a strong LOR, giving insider advice on interviews, or connecting them to key faculty.

How to Apply and Secure Placements

For international medical graduates, securing USCE is one of the most crucial steps toward building a competitive residency application.

While test scores and research productivity are vital, many residency program directors emphasize that hands-on or observational clinical exposure in the United States demonstrates readiness for the American healthcare environment. It shows adaptability, familiarity with the U.S. system, and a genuine commitment to pursuing a career in this setting.

That said, the process of applying and securing clinical placements can feel overwhelming for IMGs. The landscape is competitive, decentralized, and often costly. This section provides a structured roadmap for navigating the application process, identifying the types of opportunities available, and maximizing your chances of success.

1. Understanding the Types of U.S. Clinical Experience

As discussed earlier, before diving into applications, it's important to recognize the categories of USCE, like observerships, externships, electives, research fellowships or positions, or clerkships.

Understanding which category applies to you (student vs. graduate) is the first filter in deciding where and how to apply.

2. Timing the Application

Timing is critical. Clinical experience is most valuable within one or two years of residency application, as program directors prefer recent exposure. Older experiences may still carry weight but may not satisfy requirements for "recent U.S. experience" (often defined as within the past two to three years).

- **For students:** Start planning in your third or fourth year of medical school. Many U.S. universities require applications six to twelve months in advance.
- **For graduates:** Begin as soon as possible, keeping in mind visa requirements, credentialing, and program deadlines.

3. Researching Programs and Opportunities

There is no single centralized system for securing clinical experience. Instead, IMGs must research across multiple sources:

- **University-based electives and observerships:** Many U.S. medical schools accept international students for electives, though eligibility criteria vary. Examples include Harvard, Johns Hopkins, and Mayo Clinic, but these are extremely competitive.
- **IMG-focused programs:** Some hospitals and institutions explicitly run programs for IMGs (e.g., Cleveland Clinic, Mount Sinai).

- **Private agencies:** Companies such as AMO (American Medical Opportunities), FMG Portal, and others connect IMGs to preceptors. While convenient, these are fee-based and should be vetted carefully for legitimacy.
- **Networking-based placements:** Sometimes opportunities arise via direct connections with attendings, alumni, or local communities.
- **Research postings:** Even if research is the primary role, many labs allow exposure to clinics or interaction with physician-scientists.

Key tip: Always cross-check reviews from past IMGs before committing, especially when paying for a placement.

4. Eligibility Requirements

Each program has specific requirements, but common ones include:

- Student status, many electives are open only to students enrolled in a medical school (not graduates).
- Transcripts and dean's letter, official documents to confirm standing.
- Immunization records, proof of vaccinations such as MMR, varicella, hepatitis B, influenza, and TB testing.
- Health insurance, required for participation.

- Background checks or drug screening, increasingly standard for hospital-based programs.
- English proficiency, TOEFL or proof of proficiency may be requested.

5. Visa Considerations

Visa status plays a major role in planning. For clinical electives, many programs accept students on a B-1/B-2 visa, while others may require J-1 or even F-1 status if affiliated with an academic exchange. Graduates must be particularly careful, as observerships often specify acceptable visa categories.

Tip: Always clarify visa requirements with the hosting institution before applying. Attempting to participate under the wrong visa can lead to complications at the border or even long-term entry bans.

6. Application Materials

Most institutions will require a combination of:

- Curriculum vitae (CV) tailored to highlight medical training, research, and clinical interests.
- Personal statement explaining your motivation for U.S. clinical exposure and career goals.
- Letters of recommendation from home-country professors or physicians (for electives).
- Medical school documents, transcripts, dean's letter, diploma (if graduated).

- Proof of immunizations and insurance.

Private agencies may streamline requirements, but university-affiliated programs often follow strict formalities.

7. Cost Considerations

USCE is rarely free. Costs can include:

- Application fees, often \$50 to \$500.
- Tuition or rotation fees, some electives cost \$1,000 to \$3,500 per month.
- Living expenses, accommodation, food, and transportation.
- Visa and travel costs.

IMGs should budget realistically, as underfunding can jeopardize participation.

8. Strategies to Maximize Success

- Apply early, many top programs fill slots a year in advance.
- Cast a wide net, apply to multiple institutions simultaneously.
- Polish your CV and personal statement, highlight clinical interest areas relevant to U.S. practice.
- Leverage alumni networks, reach out to senior IMGs from your country who have successfully rotated.
- Stay flexible, even community hospitals or smaller clinics can provide meaningful U.S. experience and LORs.

Documentation and Letters of Recommendation

Letters of recommendation (LORs) are one of the most critical outputs of U.S. clinical experience. According to NRMP Program Director Surveys, LORs rank among the top factors influencing residency interview offers. Well-written, personalized letters from U.S. physicians can significantly enhance an IMG's credibility.

1. Importance of Documentation

Strong documentation serves two purposes:

1. **Proof of experience:** Many residency programs require evidence of clinical participation. Certificates or evaluation forms from the host institution are valuable.
2. **Supportive evaluation:** Narrative assessments from U.S. physicians provide insights into your clinical ability, adaptability, and communication skills.

2. Types of Letters of Recommendation

- **Standard LORs:** Written by U.S. physicians you worked with.
- **Departmental or chair's letter:** Sometimes required by specific specialties (such as internal medicine).
- **Research letters:** From supervisors in academic or lab settings. These can supplement but not replace clinical LORs.
- **Home-country letters:** Useful, but typically secondary to U.S.-based letters.

3. How to Earn a Strong LOR

- Show initiative, be punctual, enthusiastic, and proactive.
- Engage in discussions, demonstrate clinical reasoning and evidence-based knowledge.
- Communicate clearly, residency programs look for teamwork and patient communication skills.
- Request early, ask for a letter while impressions are fresh. Provide your CV and personal statement to help your preceptor.
- Target specialty alignment, seek LORs from physicians in the specialty you intend to apply for.

4. Logistics of Submitting LORs

- LORs are uploaded through ERAS (Electronic Residency Application Service). IMGs cannot upload letters themselves; instead, physicians or their staff must upload directly.
- Always provide your letter writer with detailed instructions and deadlines.
- Aim for three or four strong U.S. LORs, supplemented by others if needed.

5. Common Pitfalls

- Generic letters, "To whom it may concern" letters without detail carry little weight.

- Too many home-country letters, programs may view these as less relevant.
- Late requests, preceptors may not have time to write meaningful evaluations if rushed.
- Unaligned specialty letters, a letter from a pediatrician may not help if you're applying for surgery.

6. Beyond Letters, Documenting Professional Growth

In addition to LORs, IMGs should keep copies of:

- Certificates of completion.
- Performance evaluations.
- Research abstracts or posters presented during U.S. rotations.

These documents provide additional material for your residency application and future credentialing.

Types of Letters of Recommendation Clinical LORs

- Written by U.S. physicians who supervised the IMG in a clinical setting.
- These are the most valuable type of LORs for residency applications.

Specialty-Specific LORs

- From physicians in the specialty the IMG is applying to (such as internal medicine or surgery).
- Strongly preferred by most residency programs.

Departmental or Chair's Letters

- Some institutions require a letter from the department chair (common in surgery, internal medicine, and pediatrics).
- These letters may summarize multiple evaluations but carry institutional authority.

Research LORs

- Written by a principal investigator or supervisor in research.
- Useful for academic credibility but should supplement, not replace, clinical letters.

Home-Country Letters

- From professors or supervisors abroad.
- These can add depth but are generally secondary to U.S.-based letters.

How Many Letters Are Needed?

ERAS allows applicants to submit up to four LORs per program. Most IMGs should aim for three strong U.S. clinical LORs, ideally specialty-specific, supplemented by one additional letter (which could be research-based or from the home country).

How to Earn a Strong Letter of Recommendation

Building Rapport with Preceptors

To secure a meaningful letter, IMGs must go beyond passive observation. Preceptors are more likely to write strong letters if they:

- See consistent professionalism and punctuality.

- Witness active engagement in discussions and clinical reasoning.
- Observe compassionate patient interactions.
- Recognize initiative, such as reviewing cases beforehand or asking thoughtful questions.

Demonstrating Clinical Knowledge

IMGs should prepare thoroughly before rotations, reviewing common cases in the specialty. Confidence and competence during presentations and discussions can leave a strong impression on attendings.

Communication and Teamwork

Residency programs value applicants who can integrate seamlessly into multidisciplinary teams. Being respectful to nurses, allied health staff, and peers is as important as impressing attendings.

Asking for the Letter

The timing and manner of the request matter:

- Ask early, near the end of the rotation, while impressions are fresh.
- Be direct but polite, "Dr. X, I greatly appreciated the opportunity to work with you. Would you feel comfortable supporting my residency application with a strong letter of recommendation?"

- Provide materials, share your CV, personal statement, and a summary of your career goals to help your preceptor write a targeted letter.

Specialty Alignment

Whenever possible, secure LORs from the specialty you are applying to. For example, an applicant to internal medicine should prioritize letters from internists or subspecialists, rather than from unrelated fields.

Writing and Logistics of LORs ERAS Requirements

- Applicants cannot upload letters themselves.
- Preceptors must submit directly through the ERAS Letter of Recommendation Portal (LoRP).
- IMGs assign letters to specific programs within ERAS after submission.

Formatting Strong LORs

While IMGs cannot control the exact content of letters, providing guidance to letter writers can help. A strong LOR generally includes:

1. Introduction, how the writer knows the applicant and for how long.
2. Clinical evaluation, description of the applicant's clinical skills, reasoning, and decision-making.
3. Professional traits, teamwork, reliability, and communication.

4. Comparisons, placing the applicant in context ("among the top 10% of trainees I have worked with").
5. Endorsement, a clear, strong statement of support.

Confidentiality

Residency programs prefer confidential letters. Applicants should waive the right to view their LORs when generating ERAS requests, as non-confidential letters are viewed less favorably.

Common Pitfalls in LORs

1. Generic or vague letters, such as "hardworking," without examples.
2. Weak endorsements, for example, "I recommend without reservation" is weaker than "I give my highest recommendation."
3. Unrelated specialty, a dermatology LOR adds little value if applying to pediatrics.
4. Late submissions, letters arriving after ERAS deadlines can jeopardize interview chances.
5. Over-reliance on home-country letters, U.S.-based letters are essential.

Additional Documentation Beyond LORs

Residency applications also benefit from:

- Certificates of completion from electives, externships, or observerships.
- Performance evaluations that provide structured feedback.
- Research abstracts or publications resulting from U.S. rotations.
- Continuing Medical Education (CME) certificates obtained during U.S. training.

Maintaining an organized portfolio ensures easy access to supporting documents when programs request verification.

Best Practices for IMGs

- Aim for three to four U.S. clinical LORs aligned with your specialty.
- Request letters early and politely, providing a CV and a personal statement.
- Prioritize quality and detail over quantity.
- Maintain organized records of certificates and evaluations.
- Avoid generic or irrelevant letters.

Conclusion

For international medical graduates, documentation and letters of recommendation form the backbone of a competitive residency application. While USMLE scores may open the door, strong LORs and proof of meaningful U.S. clinical experience demonstrate readiness for the realities of American residency training.

A well-documented clinical portfolio, anchored by compelling, detailed, and specialty-specific letters of recommendation, can transform an applicant's chances of success. Conversely, weak or poorly managed letters can undermine even the strongest academic credentials.

By approaching documentation strategically, engaging actively during clinical experiences, and cultivating supportive relationships with U.S. physicians, IMGs can secure the endorsements needed to cross the threshold from abroad to MD in the United States.

Chapter 6:
Research and Publications

When you are applying for residency as an International Medical Graduate (IMG) in the U.S., your academic credentials (medical school performance, USMLE scores, clinical rotations, letters of recommendation) are extremely important. However, in this competitive field, research and publications can make a huge difference between being one among many and being remembered.

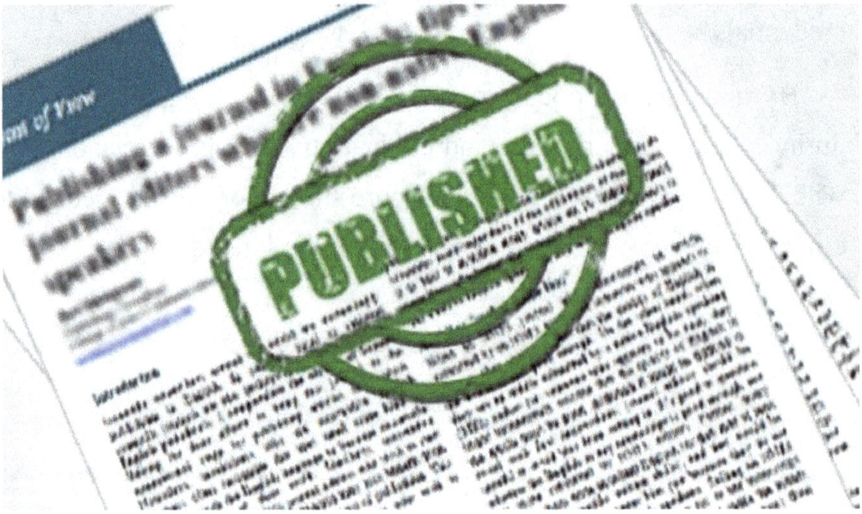

This chapter will explore why research matters, what types of research IMGs can pursue, how to approach mentors or labs, how to write abstracts, posters, and papers, and how to balance research with the heavy load of exam preparation.

The Role of Research in Strengthening Residency Applications

Let's start with why research is valuable. The U.S. residency match process is fiercely competitive, especially for IMGs. According to data, while U.S. MD graduates often match at very high rates (90-plus percent in many specialties), IMGs' match rates are lower.

But among successful IMG applicants, those with research experience often perform better in interviews, earn stronger letters of recommendation, show greater familiarity with U.S. academic culture, and sometimes overcome weaker parts of their application.

Although research alone will not entirely compensate for low exam scores, poor clinical evaluations, or weak letters, it can meaningfully augment an application.

Here are specific ways research helps:

- **Demonstrates academic curiosity and critical thinking.** Residency programs want residents who can read the literature, ask questions, think of improvements, and understand evidence-based medicine. Doing research shows you can do that.
- **Shows commitment to medicine beyond routine clinical duties.** It sends a message that you are willing to invest extra time, learn new skills (statistics, writing, presentation), and engage in teamwork in academia.

- **Creates opportunities for publications, posters, and presentations.** All of these are components of a strong CV. A publication, even in a lesser-known journal, is often more powerful than many clinical rotations alone, especially if it is original research.
- **Earns stronger letters of recommendation.** Working closely with mentors (especially U.S.-based or academic mentors) in research gives you chances for meaningful evaluations. A mentor who knows you well is in a better position to write detailed, specific, and glowing letters rather than generic ones.
- **Helps with interviews.** When interviewers ask, "Tell me about a time you contributed to research," or "What was your favorite project?", having real experience gives you concrete stories to tell. You may also be asked about methodology, interpretation of data, and ethics, all areas where practicing research helps.
- **Supports specialty choice.** If you aim for certain competitive specialties, such as dermatology, neurosurgery, plastic surgery, or interventional radiology, programs often expect more research. Even in less competitive specialties, research in your chosen field signals real interest.
- **Network and reputation.** Co-authors, mentors, and collaborators become part of your professional network. Institutions and publications are remembered. Having names of recognized labs, professors, and journals helps.

- **Home-country research counts.** If you did meaningful research in your home country, especially with publications or presentations, it still matters. Residency programs understand that IMGs may have fewer opportunities. However, U.S.-based research is often seen as more relevant because of familiarity with local systems, IRB processes, patient populations, and expectations.
- Some studies have described how IMGs who dedicate research years improve their match chances and have shown that many IMGs who matched into neurosurgery had prior research experience.
- In summary, research is not optional if you want to stand out. It is an essential distinguishing factor.

Opportunities for IMGs: Types of Research

Having established why research matters, let's consider what kinds of research are possible and how IMGs can find and use them.

There are broadly three or four types of research:

- Clinical research
- Bench (basic science or translational) research
- Public health, epidemiology, or global health
- Quality improvement, health systems, or implementation science

Each has its own strengths, feasibility, and relevance based on your situation.

Clinical Research

Clinical research often involves patient populations, clinical trials, retrospective chart reviews, case reports and case series, cohort studies, and similar designs. For IMGs, clinical research is valuable because:

- It often translates more directly to patient care, which residency programs value.
- It exposes you to IRB (Institutional Review Board) processes, patient consent, data handling, obtaining clinical data, and interacting with patients, all of which are relevant to clinical training.

Challenges may include access to clinical data, which often requires affiliation with hospitals or clinics in the U.S. or your home country, with appropriate oversight. If you are already doing electives or observerships, you might ask if you can help with any ongoing clinical research.

Bench / Basic Science / Translational Research

This involves lab work, experiments, animal models, molecular biology, biochemistry, sometimes translational work (bench to bedside), and possibly genomics.

The upside is that it is often highly regarded, especially in academic specialties. It can lead to very impactful publications. However, it can also be more resource-intensive, requiring specialized labs, equipment, and sometimes more time, as well as mentorship.

Many IMGs find bench research challenging because securing positions in lab groups in the U.S. as a non-citizen or before completing all credentials can be more difficult. Nevertheless, for those who can access it, bench research adds a strong component.

Public Health / Epidemiology / Global Health

If your interest lies there, this is a highly viable path. Projects can include epidemiological data analyses, disease prevalence or risk factor studies, community health initiatives, global health projects crossing borders, and health policy development.

These often allow remote collaboration, secondary data usage, analysis of public data sets, and sometimes less dependence on expensive bench infrastructure. It is particularly helpful if you have language skills or ties to regions outside the U.S.

Quality Improvement (QI) / Health Systems Science

These are increasingly valued by U.S. residency programs. Hospitals and clinics often run QI projects under ACGME frameworks. Projects may involve process improvements, patient safety, patient satisfaction, electronic medical record (EMR) workflows, cost savings, and similar initiatives.

For IMGs, especially those with U.S. clinical exposure (observerships, externships, or volunteer roles), participating in QI adds a dimension to your experience, showing you can think critically about system challenges.

Where and How to Find Opportunities

- In academic hospitals or large centers of your home country, even if the lab equipment is less advanced, meaningful clinical or epidemiologic projects can be completed. Publications and abstracts still matter.
- U.S. institutions, during electives, observerships, remote collaboration, or formal research fellowships.
- Summer research programs or scholarship programs (if you are a student) or post-graduate research fellowships.
- Online resources, platforms, or organizations that connect IMGs to research positions.
- NIH and government-funded positions (if eligible), or non-profit or global health organizations that allow international collaborations.
- Volunteer assistant roles in labs or with professors in universities, even if unpaid, if they lead to publications, presentations, or concrete output.
- Research databases and job boards specifically oriented toward IMGs or unmatched physicians, which often list clinical research positions.

How to Approach Professors, Labs, and Hospitals

Securing a research position often depends on how well you reach out and present yourself. For many IMGs, this part is daunting. However, with strategy, persistence, and professionalism, it is doable.

Identify What You Want

First, decide on:

- The specialty or field you are most interested in.
- Whether you prefer clinical, public health, bench, or QI research.
- The amount of time you can commit (weeks, months, a year, part-time remote, or full-time on-site).
- Whether you need paid work or are comfortable with volunteer work.

Finding Potential Mentors or Labs

- Use PubMed or Google Scholar to find researchers in your field of interest. Review recent papers, identify corresponding authors, and assess whether they are active in that domain.
- Explore faculty pages at U.S. medical schools or large hospitals, including specialty departments. International academic institutions may also have U.S.-trained faculty with connections.
- Identify labs or departments with ongoing projects aligned with your interests. Some labs advertise research assistant or volunteer positions on their websites.

- Alumni or contacts who have already matched as IMGs or are doing research can be helpful sources of leads.
- Use research opportunity aggregators or databases designed for IMGs.

Crafting the Outreach Email

Your email to a professor, principal investigator (PI), or lab director should be concise, friendly, professional, and demonstrate that you have done your homework.

Include in your email:

- A short introduction: who you are, where you studied, whether you have ECFMG certification (if applicable), your clinical exposure, and your current stage in the IMG journey.
- Your research interest: mention a recent paper they published or a project of theirs you would like to contribute to.
- What you offer: your skills (data entry, literature review, statistics, lab work, coding), your availability, and whether you can work remotely or need to be on-site.
- What you want: clarify whether you are seeking a volunteer research assistant role, authorship, poster preparation, or manuscript collaboration.
  • Attach your CV (research-formatted if possible), any previous publications or abstracts, relevant test scores or certifications (such as USMLE or ECFMG), and suggest possible times for a meeting or call if appropriate.

- Be polite, express gratitude, and avoid generic language. Make the email specific.

Negotiating Terms and Getting Commitment

- Once a PI shows interest, clarify expectations, including deliverables (abstract, poster, manuscript), timelines, specific tasks, mentorship structure, and meeting frequency.
- Clarify authorship expectations upfront if relevant. If you plan to analyze data, run experiments, and write sections, authorship should be discussed clearly.
- Confirm logistical matters such as IRB or ethics oversight, required training (such as CITI), hospital clearance, and access to data or EMR systems.
- Understand whether funding or a stipend is available. Many positions are volunteer or unpaid, especially for remote or academic roles.

Remote and Volunteer Positions

- Many U.S. labs are open to remote literature reviews, data analysis, systematic reviews, and meta-analyses. These tasks can often be completed from abroad if time zones permit.
- Volunteer work without payment can still be extremely valuable if it leads to publications, authorship, or strong letters of recommendation.

- During COVID-19, remote and virtual research collaborations expanded, and many PIs remain open to remote participation for non-lab tasks.

Using Your Home Country as a Resource

As many IMGs are still in their home country, you can conduct meaningful clinical, epidemiologic, or global health research locally.

Identify academic teaching hospitals, research organizations, non-profits, or public health departments. Seek mentors who have ties to international research or who publish in internationally indexed journals. Aim to publish in internationally recognized journals or present at international conferences, either virtually or in person.

Even retrospective chart reviews, audits, or epidemiologic surveys conducted at your local hospital can become publishable work if the methodology is sound.

Examples and Anecdotes

There are IMGs who have secured clinical research coordinator positions in U.S. hospitals, sometimes as non-U.S. citizens or visa-requiring individuals. One IMG reported that working as a CRC helped them obtain multiple publications, strengthen letters of recommendation, and match successfully.

Another common pattern is for an IMG in their home country to begin with small retrospective studies or case reports, learn to analyze data, write abstracts, and gradually collaborate with international mentors, sometimes transitioning into research roles in the U.S. or remote collaborator positions.

Writing Abstracts, Posters, and Papers

Having research experience is one side; presenting it well is just as important. This section deals with how to prepare abstracts, posters, and manuscripts, and how to understand the publication process.

Abstracts and Posters

Abstracts are short summaries of research designs, results, and conclusions. They are used for conference submissions or sometimes included in applications. Posters are visual presentations summarizing your research, typically displayed at meetings or conferences.

Tips to write abstracts:

- Keep abstracts concise and clear. Include background, objectives, methods, results, and conclusions (if results are available). If results are preliminary or ongoing, you can present what you have, but be honest.
- Use clear language: avoid excessive jargon, define terms, and ensure your question, method, and findings are understandable.
- Grant structure: always include the "why" (why this matters), "how" (how you did it), "what you found," and "what it implies."

- Before submitting to a conference, check deadlines, formatting requirements, word or character limits, and whether the meeting allows abstracts from international collaborators or IMGs.
- Posters: visually appealing layout matters. Use graphs and tables, bullet summaries, and avoid dense text. Practice explaining your poster to non-experts, as you may need to discuss it with a variety of people at conferences.
- If presenting at a conference, prepare a short "elevator pitch" for the poster, a one- to two-minute summary, and be ready for questions.

Manuscripts and Publications

Publishing is often the most time-consuming part of research in terms of writing, revisions, and peer review, but it provides the most substantial evidence of research productivity.

Steps and tips:

1. **Designing the study well before collecting data.** A poorly designed study can generate data but weak conclusions. Key tools include defining hypotheses, identifying variables, ensuring an adequate sample size, considering potential biases, and planning statistical analyses.

2. **Literature review.** Before you begin, read widely. Know what has been done and what gaps exist. This helps you define novel contributions and justify your study.

Writing:

3. **Title and abstract:** These are often the first elements reviewers and readers see. Make them compelling and accurate.

   Introduction: Establish background, the gap in knowledge, and the purpose of the study.

   Methods: Clearly describe how data were collected or experiments conducted. Include statistical tools, ethical considerations, setting, inclusion and exclusion criteria, and other relevant details.

   Results: Use appropriate tables and figures. Be precise and avoid overinterpretation.

   Discussion: Interpret results, discuss limitations, compare findings with prior literature, and suggest implications and future directions.

   Conclusion: Briefly state the main message; sometimes include suggestions or recommendations.

4. **Authorship and ethics:** Be clear about who did what. Avoid honorary authorship. Use guidelines such as ICMJE to understand authorship criteria. Ensure IRB or ethics approval if human subjects or data are involved, and maintain proper consent procedures.

5. **Peer review and revision:** After submitting to a journal, you will likely receive reviewer comments. Respond politely and

constructively, and be prepared to revise your manuscript. Reviewers may request additional analyses, clarification, or reformatting. Be patient, as this process can take several months.

6. **Choosing a journal:** Consider impact factor, audience, indexing, open access versus subscription, and publication fees. Sometimes it is better to aim for a more modest journal with a higher likelihood of acceptance than to face repeated rejections from top-tier journals. For IMGs, having something published is often better than waiting for a perfect placement.

7. **Preprint servers:** In some fields, preprints have grown in acceptability and allow early dissemination. However, some journals do not accept manuscripts that have been posted as preprints, or accept them only under certain conditions. Always check journal policies beforehand.

8. **Presentations and conferences:** Presenting as a poster or oral presentation increases visibility and provides material to discuss during interviews. Even virtual conferences count. Conference abstracts may also appear in proceedings, which adds to your CV.

9. **Track your work:** Maintain a database or spreadsheet of all your projects, including title, status (planning, data collection, analysis, writing, submitted, accepted, published), your role,

and expected dates. This aids time management and follow-up and prevents projects from being forgotten.

Common Pitfalls and How to Avoid Them

- Doing too many small, disjointed projects with no output. It is better to complete one or two projects well and publish them.
- Undertaking projects without mentorship or without clarity regarding tasks, authorship, and expectations.
- Poor study design, including failure to consider bias, sample size, or a statistical plan.
- Delays in IRB approval, data access, or writing. Avoid overpromising; plan buffer time instead.
- Poor journal selection, including overly ambitious targets or predatory journals. Ensure journals are legitimate, indexed, and peer-reviewed.
- Poor documentation or data organization, leading to lost work or unclear contributions.

Balancing Research with Exam Preparation and Clinical Work

One of the biggest challenges for IMGs is time. You will likely be preparing for USMLE Step exams, arranging clinical rotations or U.S. clinical experience, securing letters of recommendation, and conducting research. Managing all of these well can feel overwhelming.

Here is how to balance them.

Planning and Time Management

- Start early. If you are still a medical student, aim to gain research experience in your early years. Even small projects during summers or lighter clinical periods can accumulate meaningfully.
- Set realistic research goals. Estimate how many hours per week you can commit without compromising exam preparation or clinical responsibilities.
- Use tools such as calendars, task trackers, and spreadsheets. Break project timelines into phases: idea → IRB or ethics approval → data collection → analysis → writing → submission.
- Prioritize wisely. In some specialties, exam scores carry more weight than research. Do not let research compromise your USMLE performance.

Integrating Research into Other Activities

- Combine research with electives or observerships. For example, during an internal medicine rotation, ask whether there are departmental projects you can assist with.
- Use remote or data-driven projects when your clinical schedule is tight, such as retrospective chart reviews, systematic reviews, meta-analyses, or public database analyses.

- Use breaks or off-periods (summer, holidays) for intensive research work.
- Collaborate with other students or IMGs. Sharing workload (data collection, literature review) can make larger projects feasible.

Maintaining Quality While Managing Load

- Never compromise quality for quantity. One strong publication or poster with clear involvement and mentorship outweighs multiple low-quality outputs.
- Be honest about your availability. Incomplete or abandoned projects are more damaging than having fewer completed ones.
- If needed, pause or slow projects rather than abandoning them abruptly. Document your contributions so they remain part of your experience.
- Keep exam preparation in focus. Define periods when research takes a back seat (such as immediately before exams), then resume afterward.

Putting It All Together: Strategy and Examples

To illustrate how this works in practice, here are hypothetical or real-based scenarios of IMGs using research to strengthen their applications, with timelines and trade-offs.

Scenario 1: Medical Student in Home Country

Raj is in his third year at a medical school in India and plans to apply for U.S. residency in two years.

In his spare time, he joins a retrospective chart review of diabetic foot ulcers at a large teaching hospital. He also learns statistics through free online courses and becomes comfortable with SPSS and R. He obtains IRB approval, collects data, writes a manuscript, and submits it to a journal.

He presents the data as a poster at a national conference in his country and later at an international conference (virtually). Meanwhile, he studies for Step 1 and scores well. He uses the publication and poster in his ERAS application and receives strong letters of recommendation from his mentor.

When applying, his application appears balanced: strong Step 1 score, clinical electives, and a publication. He matches into internal medicine.

Scenario 2: Unmatched or Recently Graduated IMG in the U.S.

Maria, an IMG who recently passed USMLE Step 2 CK, is completing observerships in the U.S. She seeks an unpaid clinical research coordinator position in a hospital research department.

She finds a remote collaboration opportunity with a U.S. professor who allows literature reviews and data abstraction from existing patient charts. She manages two projects: one retrospective study and one systematic review. She submits both for publication; one is accepted, and she also presents a poster.

Simultaneously, she continues preparing for Step 3 and other licensing requirements while maintaining active clinical exposure. This strengthens her CV enough to secure interviews in her chosen specialty.

Scenario 3: Specializing and Bench Research

Ahmed is a research-oriented IMG aspiring to neurosurgery. He secures an unpaid bench research fellowship in the U.S., working in neuro-oncology. He gains experience with animal models, molecular techniques, and translational research.

After 9 to 12 months, he has a first-author manuscript and has contributed to two additional papers. His bench research is supported by strong board exam scores and a CV showing both clinical observerships and research productivity. While neurosurgery remains highly competitive, his research improves his interview opportunities and recognition.

These examples highlight trade-offs: time invested in research reduces time for rest or exam preparation. However, when planned strategically, these sacrifices often pay off.

Action Plan: What You Should Do Now

To make the most of this information, here is a suggested action plan tailored to your timeline, whether you are one to two years from applying or closer.

1. **Assess your current situation.** What research experience do you already have? What type of research do you want (clinical, bench, public health)? How much time can you commit over the next 6 to 12 months? What specialty are you targeting?

2. **Acquire basic tools and skills early**, including:

- Basic statistical concepts (mean, median, standard deviation, hypothesis testing, p-values, confidence intervals)
- Use of statistical software (SPSS, R, Stata, Excel)
- Literature search tools (PubMed, Google Scholar, Ovid)
- Citation and reference managers (EndNote, Zotero, Mendeley)
- Scientific writing skills, focusing on clarity and structure

3. **Find mentors and opportunities.** Start with your existing network: professors, alumni, senior students, and research centers in your city or country. Reach out to U.S. mentors by email when possible. Use research opportunity databases and explore remote collaboration options.

4. **Plan projects strategically.** Aim for a mix of shorter projects (case reports, retrospective studies) that yield quicker results and one larger project (systematic review, bench research, or cohort study) with higher long-term value.

5. **Document everything.** Track your roles, timelines, outputs, and outcomes. This simplifies CV writing, personal statements, and interview preparation.

6. **Prepare publications and presentations early.** Do not wait until deadlines approach.

7. **Balance with exam preparation.** Schedule research around board exams and reduce workload as exams approach. Remember that exam scores are often non-negotiable.

8. **Refine and revise.** Be open to feedback on abstracts and manuscripts. Learn from mentors, peer reviewers, and colleagues.

Conclusion

Research and publications are not optional extras for IMGs; they are essential components of a competitive U.S. residency application.

When pursued thoughtfully, research demonstrates academic seriousness and capability, strengthens letters of recommendation, provides interview talking points, and adds credibility, especially when other areas of the application have limitations.

This does not mean doing everything. The goal is not perfection, but strategic, high-quality contributions aligned with your specialty interests and timeline. If you start early, make informed choices, seek strong mentorship, and manage your time wisely, research can be both feasible and highly rewarding.

Chapter 7:
Applying to Residency Programs

Applying to U.S. residency programs is perhaps the most critical phase of your journey as an International Medical Graduate. It requires careful planning, excellent documentation, and an understanding of how the system works.

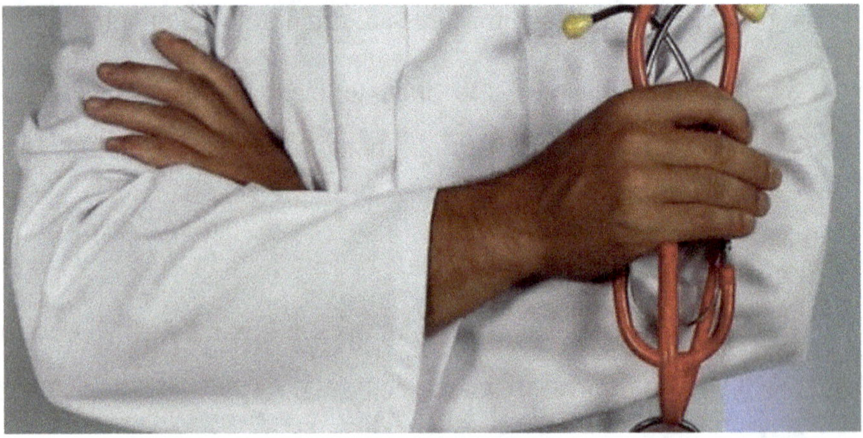

In this chapter, we will cover how ERAS works, how to craft a compelling personal statement, the right format for your CV, the importance of letters of recommendation and MSPEs, the competitiveness of different specialties (especially for IMGs), and strategies to boost your chances, especially via community programs, smaller hospitals, or other less traditional but effective pathways.

The ERAS Application System Explained

ERAS stands for the Electronic Residency Application Service. It is the centralized online system through which applicants submit their applications and supporting documents to U.S. residency programs.

For IMGs, ERAS is managed via ECFMG (Educational Commission for Foreign Medical Graduates). Your documents, including transcripts, letters of recommendation (LORs), and proof of medical credentials, are uploaded, verified, and then sent to all the programs you apply to through ERAS.

Key Components of ERAS

The Electronic Residency Application Service is the central platform used by medical graduates to apply for residency programs in the United States.

For international medical graduates (IMGs), understanding its key components is essential to avoid delays or mistakes that could cost valuable opportunities. While the system may appear overwhelming at first, breaking it down into its main parts makes the process much more manageable.

MyERAS Portal

At the heart of the system is the MyERAS portal, which functions as your personal dashboard. This is where you will spend the most time, entering all of the information that residency programs will review.

You'll fill in personal details, examination scores such as USMLE Step 1, Step 2 CK, and Step 3 (if applicable), as well as details about your medical education, hospital or clinical experiences, and any observerships or externships.

In addition, you'll record research projects, publications, volunteer experiences, and other accomplishments.

Think of MyERAS as your professional showcase, it's essentially a highly structured résumé that allows programs to compare applicants side by side. Accuracy and attention to detail here are crucial because errors or omissions could reflect poorly on your application.

Supporting Documents

Your application is only as strong as the documents that support it. These include your medical school transcript, the Medical Student Performance Evaluation (MSPE, often called a Dean's Letter), and your proof of ECFMG certification for IMGs. For international graduates, ECFMG oversees the process of verifying and uploading these documents into the system.

Letters of recommendation are also vital; these should ideally come from U.S. physicians you have worked with during rotations, observerships, or research.

Some programs may request a professional photograph to be included in your file. Each document must be submitted according to strict specifications, and since ECFMG is the intermediary for IMGs, their processing times must also be factored in. Planning ahead ensures everything is uploaded before deadlines.

ERAS Token from ECFMG

Before IMGs can even log in to MyERAS, they need an ERAS token, which is issued by the Educational Commission for Foreign Medical Graduates (ECFMG). This token acts as your unique identifier in the system and links your documents with your application.

Tokens are usually available each spring, and it's important to request one as soon as they become available. Without this step, you cannot register or begin your application.

Program Documents and Application

Once the basics are complete, the next step is choosing the programs to which you want to apply. Within MyERAS, you'll find detailed application sections about your education, clinical and research experiences, skills, honors, and extracurricular activities.

Each program may also include program-specific requirements or supplemental questions.

For instance, some may ask you to complete an additional form or submit specific essays about your interest in their institution. Carefully review each program's requirements so nothing is missed.

Submission and Transmission Deadlines

Finally, deadlines are among the most critical components of ERAS. The system has specific dates for when applications open, when supporting documents must be uploaded, and when programs begin downloading and reviewing applications.

For IMGs, the ECFMG publishes a detailed timeline guide to help applicants track these dates. Missing a deadline for documents, such as a transcript or recommendation letter, can result in your application not being considered, even if the rest of your materials were submitted on time.

Because residency is highly competitive, it's always best to have everything prepared and uploaded well before the final dates.

In short, ERAS is a structured but complex system. Understanding its key components, MyERAS, supporting documents, tokens, program applications, and deadlines, can help you navigate it confidently and avoid last-minute stress. By organizing your materials early and carefully following instructions, you'll ensure that your application is complete and ready for review when programs begin evaluating candidates.

ERAS for IMGs: Special Considerations

For international medical graduates, applying to U.S. residency programs through the ERAS involves additional layers of preparation compared to U.S. medical students. The system itself is the same, but IMGs must meet specific requirements related to verification, certification, and document submission that are overseen by the ECFMG.

Understanding these special considerations early on will save you stress and ensure that your application is not delayed.

Credential Verification

One of the first steps for IMGs is ensuring that their academic credentials, such as their medical degree and transcripts, are properly verified.

Unlike U.S. graduates, who already have standardized reporting systems in place, IMGs often face extra requirements. For example, if your documents are not in English, they must be translated by an approved service.

Some documents may also require notarization to prove authenticity. These steps can take weeks or even months, depending on your country's regulations and your medical school's responsiveness. Because of this, IMGs should start the credential verification process as early as possible.

The ECFMG Status Report

A key document that residency programs will see in your ERAS application is the ECFMG Status Report.

This report verifies that you are certified by ECFMG or shows that your certification is still in progress. It also includes the dates when you passed your USMLE exams.

Programs rely on this report to confirm your eligibility, so it's essential that your certification status is up to date. If you are still waiting on a required exam, programs will be able to see that as well. For many programs, incomplete certification can be a red flag, so you should aim to have your requirements fulfilled well before applications open.

MSPE / Dean's Letter Equivalents

In the United States, medical schools issue a standardized Medical Student Performance Evaluation (MSPE), also known as the Dean's Letter, which provides a narrative assessment of a student's academic performance, professionalism, and clinical skills.

IMGs are required to submit their own equivalent. This may not always be a standard document at international schools, which means you may have to request one specifically from your dean's office.

At a minimum, the document should verify your academic standing, describe your performance during clinical years, and confirm that you graduated in good standing. Because many international schools are not used to producing this type of document, communication is key, give your school plenty of time to prepare it and be ready to provide them with examples of U.S. MSPEs if necessary.

Transcripts

Your medical school transcript is another essential part of the application. This must be submitted through your designated dean's office and verified by ECFMG.

IMGs should be aware that this process often takes longer than expected. Delays can arise due to missing signatures, incomplete records, the need for translations, or verification bottlenecks.

Since ERAS has strict submission deadlines, you should begin the process well before applications open. Many IMGs underestimate the time it can take for documents to travel from their home country, be translated, and then verified by ECFMG, sometimes several months. Hence, planning ahead here is non-negotiable.

Timeline for IMGs

The residency application timeline is the same for U.S. graduates and IMGs, but because IMGs must account for extra verification steps, starting early is even more important.

Early Summer (June/July): ERAS usually opens for applicants to begin filling out their personal details, exam scores, experiences, and uploading documents. This is the time to make sure your ECFMG token is active and that you can access the MyERAS system. IMGs should ideally have all documents in progress or already submitted to ECFMG by this point.

September: Residency programs begin receiving and reviewing applications. This is the critical milestone. If your documents are not uploaded and verified by now, many programs will not consider your application.

Fall and Winter (October–January): Interview season begins. Programs invite selected applicants to interview, and this is your opportunity to showcase yourself beyond the written application.

Late Winter (February): Rank order lists must be submitted by both applicants and programs. This step finalizes the preferences for the National Resident Matching Program (NRMP).

March (Match Day): Match results are released in mid-March, and applicants find out whether and where they have matched.

For IMGs, one of the most important timeline considerations is the deadline for document submission. Letters of recommendation, transcripts, and proof of ECFMG certification must be completed well before September, when programs begin to download applications. Programs typically review files on a rolling basis, and an incomplete file could mean your application is never seen, even if it is later completed.

In short, while the ERAS application process is the same for everyone, IMGs must handle additional steps such as credential verification, dean's letters, and ECFMG certification.

Starting early, staying organized, and anticipating delays are the keys to success. By managing these special considerations ahead of time, you can ensure that your application is complete, accurate, and ready to compete on an equal footing when programs begin reviewing candidates.

Crafting a Compelling Personal Statement

One of the components that gives you a chance to stand out beyond test scores, grades, and résumé items is your personal statement. Many residency program directors say that when many applications look similar in objective measures, the personal statement is what helps them see the person behind the paper.

What to Include

Why medicine, and more specifically, why your specialty: Personal stories work, perhaps a patient encounter, academic interest, or life experience that led you toward this specialty. Be specific. Vague statements like "I love helping people" are less powerful than "During my rotation in internal medicine, seeing Mr. Smith's case of CHF taught me …"

What makes you unique: As an IMG, you have perspectives, experiences, maybe language skills, or cultural diversity. Bring those in. If you have worked abroad, in underserved areas, or done research in resource-limited settings, these show adaptability.

Challenges you have overcome: If you had to navigate financial, systemic, or logistical hurdles to pursue your medical education, explain how that shaped you. This can be compelling.

What you aim to gain and contribute: Show that you understand the residency environment, not just what you want to get, but what you can bring (teamwork, research capability, language skills, etc.).

What to Avoid

- Being overly general or cliché.
- Focusing too much on family or non-medical reasons unless they directly connect to your journey in medicine.
- Listing your CV items instead of reflecting on them. (Your CV already shows what you did; the statement should explain why and how.)
- Errors in grammar, spelling, or tone, especially tone. It should be professional but personal.

Structure & Style Tips for Writing Your Personal Statement

When writing your residency personal statement, the way you structure your story is just as important as the content you include. A strong statement follows a natural flow that guides the reader from who you are to where you want to go, all while keeping your writing concise and engaging.

A good place to begin is with a hook, something that immediately captures attention. This might be a brief anecdote, an experience that shaped your perspective on medicine, or a meaningful insight that reveals your values. The hook does not need to be dramatic; it just needs to feel personal and genuine, something that invites the reader to keep going.

From there, move into your journey. This section should highlight the experiences that have prepared you for residency and medicine in general. You might discuss clinical rotations, research projects, volunteer work, or other moments that had a lasting impact.

The goal is to show the progression of your development, how each step helped you grow into the physician you are becoming.

Once you have established that foundation, narrow the focus to your specialty interest. Programs want to know why you are drawn to a particular field. Share what excites you about the specialty, what skills you bring that are well suited to it, and what experiences have confirmed your decision.

This section should show both passion and practicality, enthusiasm backed up by evidence from your training.

After explaining your interest in the specialty, turn toward your goals. What do you hope to accomplish in residency? What type of learning environment helps you thrive? For example, you might value close mentorship, strong teamwork, or a program with robust research opportunities.

Use this space to show programs that you have thought carefully about the kind of training you seek and the contributions you hope to make during residency.

Finally, close with a forward-looking paragraph. Here, you tie together your personal journey, your interest in the specialty, and your future aspirations. Explain how residency training fits into your broader career goals and how you hope to grow within the program.

This is also a chance to highlight how you will contribute to the residency community, through your work ethic, perspective, or dedication to patients.

In terms of length, most personal statements should be about one page single-spaced, typically around 500 to 700 words. Many programs set limits, so always check the guidelines. In this case, more is not necessarily better, clarity, focus, and authenticity matter most.

CV Formatting for U.S. Standards

A well-formatted curriculum vitae (CV) that aligns with U.S. expectations is one of the most important tools in your residency application. Programs often receive thousands of applications, and a clean, professional CV allows reviewers to quickly identify your strengths, experiences, and readiness for training.

For international medical graduates, a CV is also a way to demonstrate familiarity with U.S. standards and professionalism.

Key Sections to Include

The first section should always include contact information and licensing or certification details.

Your name, phone number, professional email address, and current address should be clear and easy to find. For IMGs, including your ECFMG certification status is important, along with your USMLE or COMLEX scores, medical school details, and graduation date.

This section reassures programs that you meet basic eligibility requirements.

Next, highlight your education. Start with your medical school and then list any additional degrees, such as an MPH, MSc, or PhD. If you completed particularly relevant or exceptional coursework, such as advanced epidemiology, public health, or biomedical research, you can briefly mention it here, though most of the focus should remain on your medical training.

The clinical experience section is one of the most crucial for IMGs. Include your rotations, electives, observerships, or internships, and provide details such as the location, dates, your role, and duties. U.S. clinical experience is especially valuable because it demonstrates your ability to work within the American healthcare system. If you have completed clerkships or observerships in the U.S., make sure these are clearly highlighted.

Your research, publications, and presentations should come next. Provide details such as the title of the project, the type of work (bench, clinical, or public health research), the journal or conference, and your co-authors. Always note your specific role in the project so reviewers understand your contribution. Using a consistent citation style, such as AMA, adds a polished and professional touch.

Another section to include is honors, awards, and scholarships. These might include Dean's List equivalents, leadership awards, or scholarships earned during your medical education. Even small recognitions help demonstrate dedication and achievement.

Residency programs also value applicants who are well-rounded, so be sure to include volunteer activities and extracurriculars. Examples might be community service, global health initiatives, mentorship roles, or leadership positions in student organizations.

These activities highlight interpersonal skills and commitment to service, qualities that matter as much as clinical ability.

Finally, add a section for skills, languages, and certifications. Mention fluency in additional languages, technical computer skills (such as using electronic health record systems), and medical or procedural skills relevant to your specialty. If you hold certifications like BLS, ACLS, or PALS, list them here.

Formatting Tips

The format of your CV should be clear and consistent. Use reverse chronological order, listing your most recent experiences first. Stick to simple, professional fonts such as Times New Roman or Arial, at 11- or 12-point size for the body text and slightly larger for headings.

Ensure there is enough white space so that the document is easy to scan quickly.

When describing roles, use bullet points, but keep them succinct. Each point should begin with a strong action verb, such as "Managed," "Conducted," "Assisted," or "Analyzed." Avoid overly long explanations. Instead, focus on impact and relevance.

Proofreading is critical. Typos, inconsistent date formats, or mixed writing styles create a negative impression. Ask several trusted mentors or colleagues to review your CV before submission.

Length

For most applicants, the CV should be around two pages. Three pages may be acceptable if you have significant research experience, multiple publications, or extensive U.S. clinical training. For many IMGs, a two- to three-page CV is considered appropriate, as long as the information is relevant and presented clearly.

In short, your residency CV should be a snapshot of your medical journey, presented in a polished, professional, and easy-to-read format. Done well, it reinforces your readiness for residency and helps your application stand out.

Importance of Letters of Recommendation and MSPEs

Letters of Recommendation (LORs) and the Medical Student Performance Evaluation, also known as the Dean's Letter, are among the few subjective components of a residency application. Unlike exam scores or transcripts, which show numbers and grades, these documents provide program directors with insight into who you are as a person, how you work in clinical settings, and how others perceive your abilities and professionalism.

When it comes to letters of recommendation, the quality of the letter matters far more than the quantity.

Ideally, your letters should come from individuals who know you well and can speak about your performance in a clinical or research environment. Supervising physicians, research mentors, clinical instructors, or preceptors are strong candidates.

Whenever possible, it is highly beneficial to secure at least one letter from someone who is based in the U.S. or who has experience working in the U.S. healthcare system, as their perspective carries additional weight with residency programs.

Three strong, specific letters are usually better than multiple generic ones.

A good recommendation should highlight not only your clinical knowledge but also your interpersonal skills, professionalism, adaptability, and teamwork. To give your letter writers the best chance to support you, provide them with ample time, ideally four to six weeks, to prepare their letters.

You should also supply them with your CV, personal statement, and reminders of specific experiences you shared with them, such as memorable cases or projects. The best letters describe how long and in what capacity the writer has known you, include concrete examples of your performance, compare you to peers when possible, and give an honest assessment of how you are likely to succeed in a U.S. residency program.

The MSPE, or Dean's Letter, serves a slightly different purpose. For U.S. medical students, the MSPE is a standardized evaluation prepared by their school, summarizing academic performance, professional attributes, and overall standing.

International medical graduates, however, may not have access to the same standardized document. Instead, IMGs typically provide an equivalent letter from their dean or academic office, outlining their academic record, class ranking or percentile, grading system, and notable professional qualities.

It is important to confirm that your medical school can provide this document and that it is submitted on time through ERAS or via the ECFMG portal, if required. Delays in uploading the MSPE or its equivalent can harm your application, as programs rely on these evaluations to compare applicants fairly. Ensuring these materials are ready, accurate, and submitted early reflects both professionalism and preparedness.

Specialty Competitiveness for IMGs

Selecting a specialty is one of the most challenging decisions international medical graduates face when applying to residency programs. Some specialties are far more competitive than others, and for IMGs, the competition can be even steeper.

Understanding match statistics and trends helps applicants make informed choices and balance ambition with practicality.

According to the 2025 Match data, U.S.-citizen IMGs had a postgraduate year one (PGY-1) match rate of approximately 67.8%, while non-U.S.-citizen IMGs matched at around 58%. Internal Medicine continues to be one of the top specialties for IMGs due to the large number of available positions and relatively higher acceptance rates. In fact, IMGs filled about 44.6% of matched first-year positions in Internal Medicine in 2025, underscoring its IMG-friendliness.

On the other hand, certain specialties are considerably more competitive. Fields such as Dermatology, Orthopedic Surgery, Plastic Surgery, Neurosurgery, Otolaryngology, and Radiology (particularly diagnostic and interventional subspecialties) have limited positions and attract top-tier candidates.

These specialties usually require very high USMLE scores, extensive research experience, and strong U.S. clinical exposure. They often favor applicants with established professional networks in the U.S. healthcare system, making it difficult for IMGs to break into the system.

By contrast, specialties such as Family Medicine, Psychiatry, Pediatrics, Pathology, and Internal Medicine are considered more IMG-friendly. These fields generally have more residency positions available and slightly lower thresholds for acceptance, although they still require solid academic and clinical performance.

Programs in these specialties are also more likely to value the diverse perspectives and resilience that IMGs bring to their training environments.

It is important to remember that competitiveness does not mean impossibility. IMGs do match into highly competitive specialties, but doing so usually requires exceptional credentials, such as top USMLE scores, multiple research publications, strong U.S. clinical experience, and outstanding letters of recommendation.

Applicants must also weigh trade-offs carefully. Choosing a specialty with fewer positions may align with your passion, but it also comes with a higher risk of not matching. That is why having a backup plan is essential. Applying to a mix of specialties or having a parallel strategy, such as targeting more IMG-friendly programs while also applying to a dream specialty, can balance ambition with realism.

Ultimately, your decision should take into account not only competitiveness but also your personal interests, desired lifestyle, and long-term career objectives. Researching where IMGs have historically matched, identifying programs open to international graduates, and being honest about your own strengths and weaknesses will help you find the right path forward.

Strategies for Increasing Chances as an IMG

The U.S. residency match process is highly competitive, and international medical graduates face unique challenges compared to their U.S. counterparts. However, with the right strategies, you can significantly improve your chances of matching. Success often comes from combining persistence with a smart, targeted approach.

Below are key strategies that can make a difference in your application journey.

Broaden Your Program List

One of the most effective tactics is to apply broadly across different types of programs and locations.

While large, urban academic centers are attractive, they often receive thousands of applications and have a smaller percentage of IMGs in their residency classes. In contrast, programs located in less urban areas or at smaller teaching hospitals may be more receptive to IMG applicants.

Community hospitals, rural programs, and institutions serving underserved populations often appreciate the diverse perspectives that IMGs bring. Casting a wide net geographically increases the likelihood of finding programs that value your unique background and contributions.

Target IMG-Friendly Specialties First

Choosing the right specialty is also essential. Some fields, such as Internal Medicine, Family Medicine, Pediatrics, Psychiatry, and Pathology, have a long track record of accepting IMGs. By contrast, specialties like Dermatology, Orthopedic Surgery, and Plastic Surgery are extremely competitive, even for U.S. graduates.

If your USMLE scores or experiences are not among the top tier, applying primarily to IMG-friendly specialties may be the most realistic path. Excelling in a less competitive residency does not limit your career; many physicians later pursue subspecialties or fellowships that align with their long-term goals.

Gain U.S. Clinical Experience

U.S. clinical experience is one of the strongest ways to make your application more appealing.

Observerships, externships, and clerkships allow you to work within the U.S. healthcare system and adapt to its norms. These experiences are valuable not only for your personal growth but also because they allow you to secure letters of recommendation from U.S. physicians. Such letters carry weight with program directors, as they provide evidence of your ability to integrate into an American clinical setting.

Strengthen Application Components

Strong academic and extracurricular credentials are another critical factor. With the transition of USMLE Step 1 to pass/fail reporting, Step 2 CK scores have become even more important for IMGs.

Aim for high performance to demonstrate your readiness for residency. Research experience, including publications, conference presentations, and poster sessions, can also set you apart, particularly if you are aiming for competitive programs.

Additionally, highlight leadership roles, teamwork, and professionalism in your clinical work, as these qualities often emerge strongly in recommendation letters.

Networking and Mentorship

Building relationships can open doors. Reach out to alumni from your medical school who have matched into U.S. residency programs, especially in your chosen specialty. They can provide valuable insights, feedback on your personal statement, or even guidance through mock interviews.

Finding a mentor in the U.S. healthcare system can be especially beneficial, as they can help identify your weaknesses and advise you on which programs might be most receptive to IMGs.

Use Program Tools and Data Wisely

Leverage data-driven resources when planning your application strategy. Tools like the AAMC's Residency Explorer and NRMP's

Charting Outcomes in the Match provide detailed statistics about program requirements, IMG percentages, and applicant characteristics.

Reviewing official program websites also helps you understand expectations regarding U.S. clinical experience, letters of recommendation, and other requirements. Targeting programs that have historically accepted IMGs increases your efficiency and improves your odds of success.

Prepare Well for Interviews

When you are invited to interviews, preparation is key. Be ready to explain your medical school training, your reasons for choosing the U.S. for residency, and how your experiences demonstrate adaptability and cultural awareness.

Many programs focus heavily on "fit," seeking candidates who will integrate seamlessly into their teams, work diligently, and uphold professionalism. Practicing common interview questions and refining your communication skills will help you stand out.

Backup and Safety Plans

Finally, always have a backup plan. Consider applying to safety specialties or programs where your application is particularly competitive. If you do not match on your first attempt, parallel paths such as a research year, pre-residency fellowship, or additional U.S. clinical experience can greatly strengthen your profile for the next cycle.

Many IMGs succeed on their second or third attempt by strategically improving their applications.

In summary, while the residency match is highly competitive, IMGs can increase their chances of success by applying broadly, choosing IMG-friendly specialties, gaining U.S. clinical experience, strengthening every part of their application, and seeking mentorship.

Combining preparation with strategy not only improves your chances of matching but also helps you build a career path that aligns with your long-term goals.

Conclusion

Applying to residency as an international medical graduate is a challenging but entirely achievable process with the right preparation and strategy. The Electronic Residency Application Service (ERAS) serves as the central platform through which your application materials are submitted and reviewed.

Ensuring that every required document is accurate, properly verified, and submitted on time is one of the most critical steps to staying competitive.

Your personal statement plays a unique role in the application because it allows programs to see beyond scores and credentials. This is your opportunity to tell your story, why you chose medicine, what shaped your specialty interests, and how your past experiences have prepared you for residency.

A well-written personal statement should be personal, reflective, and clearly focused on the specialty you are applying to. It should not only highlight what you have accomplished so far but also share what you hope to contribute and achieve during residency.

A U.S.-style curriculum vitae is another essential part of your application. Residency programs are accustomed to a clear, standardized structure that highlights your education, clinical experiences, research, skills, and volunteer work. Equally important are the letters of recommendation and the Medical Student Performance Evaluation, or its equivalent. These documents provide program directors with an outside perspective on your abilities, professionalism, and potential.

In short, success in the residency application process requires both careful preparation and smart strategy. By presenting a strong, well-organized application and aligning your goals with the realities of the U.S. residency landscape, you can position yourself for the best possible chance of securing a residency position and moving forward in your medical career.

Chapter 8:
The Interview Process

Securing an interview in the U.S. residency Match is one of the biggest milestones for International Medical Graduates. After years of study, exam preparation, and clinical rotations, the invitation to interview means your application has stood out among thousands of candidates.

Yet, being offered an interview is only half the battle, the next step is showing programs that you are not only qualified but also the right fit for their team, culture, and patients.

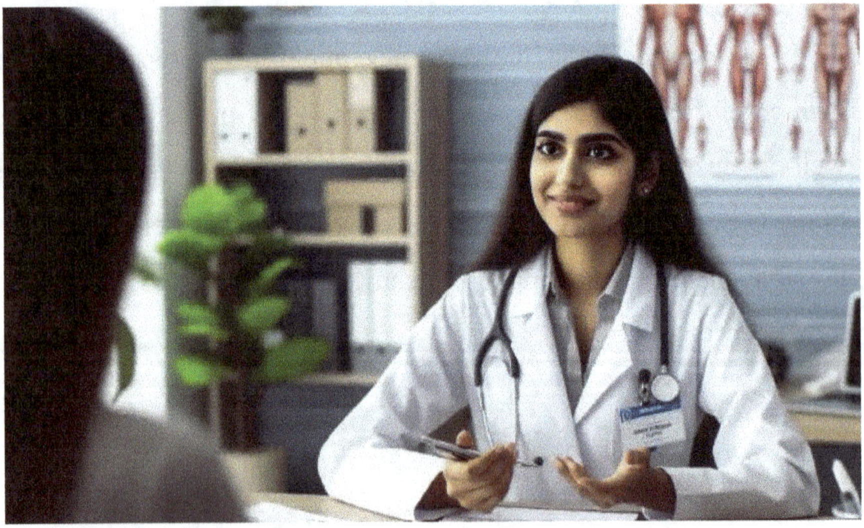

This chapter will walk you through the U.S.-style interview process in detail: how to prepare, what to expect, how to adapt to cultural nuances, and how to handle outcomes, whether positive or negative.

By the end, you'll feel equipped to confidently present yourself, manage challenges, and maximize your chances of a successful Match.

Preparing for U.S.-Style Interviews

Residency interviews are not just about verifying your qualifications. By the time you're invited, programs already know you meet their baseline criteria through your USMLE scores, MSPE, letters of recommendation, and clinical experience.

The interview is about fit, in terms of:

- Do you communicate well with patients and colleagues?
- Are you adaptable to the U.S. healthcare system?
- Can you handle the emotional and physical demands of residency?

Do your values align with the program's mission and culture?

For IMGs, interviews also help programs assess your comfort with English, professionalism in cross-cultural settings, and how well you might integrate into their team.

Researching the Program

A successful interview begins long before you log in to a virtual call or walk into a conference room. The foundation of an excellent interview lies in preparation, and the most important part of that preparation is researching each program in detail.

Residency programs are not identical; they differ in their academic focus, patient population, size, faculty interests, and culture. Interviewers expect candidates, especially international medical graduates, to demonstrate familiarity with the unique aspects of their program. This means going beyond surface-level knowledge and immersing yourself in the details that matter.

For each program, start with their official website. Review the residency curriculum, rotation schedules, and opportunities for electives or research. Take note of the program's leadership and core faculty members; reading their biographies and recent publications can help you understand their academic interests and priorities.

You may discover that a faculty member has published in your field of interest, which could become a natural talking point during the interview. Similarly, reviewing resident rosters can help you see the diversity of the cohort, the types of medical schools represented, and the potential for mentorship within the program.

Another key aspect of preparation is understanding the values of each program. Not all residencies have the same mission, and program directors want to see that you understand and respect their priorities. Some residencies emphasize care for underserved or rural populations, while others may highlight academic research, subspecialty training, or community-based medicine.

If a program clearly states that its mission is to train physicians who will serve disadvantaged populations, then your answers should reflect an alignment with this goal.

For example, you might highlight your volunteer experiences, your dedication to health equity, or your ability to adapt to working with diverse patient populations. On the other hand, if a program is affiliated with a large research institution and emphasizes scholarly productivity, you should be prepared to discuss your own research experiences, your publications, or your interest in contributing to ongoing projects.

By tailoring your preparation to the program's stated values, you not only demonstrate attentiveness but also convey genuine interest.

Equally important is researching the location where the program is based. This is a step many applicants overlook, but interviewers often appreciate it when candidates show knowledge of the city or region.
Understanding local demographics, community health needs, and even the cost of living demonstrates thoughtfulness and maturity. For instance, if the residency is located in an area with a large immigrant population, you might note how your cultural competence and multilingual abilities could help you serve that community. If the city has unique challenges, such as limited healthcare access or high rates of chronic disease, you can connect your experiences to how you would contribute to addressing those needs.

Even small details, such as mentioning awareness of the climate, transportation, or cultural attractions, can show that you are realistically considering what it would be like to live and work there.

Finally, with all of this information, you need to be able to articulate why you are drawn to that particular program. Generic statements like “I like your program because of its reputation” or “I want to work in a supportive learning environment” are too vague and could apply to nearly any residency. Instead, be prepared with specific reasons that connect your background, skills, and goals to what the program offers.

Perhaps the program’s strong emphasis on primary care aligns with your long-term plan to return to your home country and improve population health. Maybe their structured mentorship program resonates with you because you value guidance in navigating the U.S. healthcare system.

Whatever the reason, clarity and specificity will set you apart from candidates who recycle the same answers for every interview.

Preparing Your Personal Story

While researching the program is essential, an equally critical step is preparing your personal narrative.

As an IMG, your journey is often more complex than that of U.S. medical graduates. You may have studied in another country, taken additional licensing exams, sought U.S. clinical experience, and possibly faced delays or gaps in your career path. Interviewers are aware of this, and they will often ask you to summarize your background.

The challenge is condensing a diverse journey into a coherent story that resonates with U.S. program directors.

Start by crafting a clear timeline of your educational and professional path. This includes your medical school training, graduation, exam milestones (USMLE Step 1, Step 2 CK, Step 3), clinical observerships or externships in the U.S., research experiences, and any employment in healthcare.

Be transparent about gaps but frame them in a constructive light. For example, if you had a gap year while preparing for exams, emphasize the discipline and focus it required. If you worked in another healthcare-related role, explain how that broadened your perspective and made you a stronger candidate.

Having a well-structured timeline not only keeps you from stumbling during the interview but also reassures interviewers that you are reflective and organized.

Anticipating questions about your IMG status is another important preparation step. Common questions include: Why did you choose to pursue a career in the U.S.? How do you plan to adapt to the U.S. healthcare system? What challenges do you anticipate, and how will you overcome them? These questions allow program directors to assess both your motivation and adaptability. Your answers should convey intentionality. Rather than saying, "I just wanted better opportunities," you could say, "I chose the U.S. because of its emphasis on evidence-based medicine and structured residency training, which I believe will prepare me to be an excellent physician."

Instead of denying that adaptation will be difficult, you can acknowledge it while showing confidence in your ability to succeed. For instance: "I recognize that communication styles and patient expectations differ in the U.S., but my clinical rotations here have already taught me the importance of shared decision-making, and I am committed to continuing that growth."

Your strengths should also shine in your personal story. IMGs often bring unique assets that U.S. graduates may not have, such as resilience, cultural competence, and a global perspective on healthcare. These qualities are highly valued when framed positively. For example, resilience can be illustrated by explaining how you persevered through challenges such as studying for the USMLE while working part-time. Cultural competence can be highlighted through examples of caring for patients from diverse backgrounds. A global perspective might include your experience with different healthcare delivery systems, which enables you to think critically about improving patient care in the U.S.

Framing these experiences with confidence and humility will help interviewers see your IMG status as an advantage rather than a limitation.

Mock Interviews and Practice

Even the most thoroughly researched program knowledge and carefully crafted personal story will fall flat without practice. Interviews are as much about delivery as they are about content, and practicing your responses is critical to presenting yourself with clarity and confidence.

Many IMGs benefit from mock interviews, which can be done with peers, mentors, or professional services. These practice sessions give you an opportunity to test your answers in a low-stakes environment and receive constructive feedback.

One of the most important skills to practice is answering common interview questions concisely.

Many applicants make the mistake of speaking for too long, wandering off-topic, or overwhelming interviewers with excessive detail. A good rule of thumb is to keep most answers within one to two minutes. This ensures you provide enough substance without losing your audience's attention. Practicing with a timer can help you develop this skill.

Language is another area where practice pays off. Even fluent English speakers may struggle with clarity under pressure. Aim to speak slowly and clearly, avoiding filler words such as "um," "like," or "you know."

At the same time, avoid using overly technical jargon unless the context demands it. Interviews are conversations, not oral exams, and program directors are evaluating your communication skills as much as your medical knowledge.

Behavioral questions are increasingly common in residency interviews, and practicing for them requires a structured approach. These questions often begin with prompts like "Tell me about a time when..." or "Describe a situation where you..."

The STAR method, Situation, Task, Action, Result, is an effective framework for answering.

For example, if asked about a time you worked in a team, you could briefly describe the situation (a busy inpatient service), outline your role (task), explain what you did (action), and conclude with the positive outcome (result). Practicing with this structure ensures your answers are clear, organized, and memorable.

Through consistent mock interviews, you can refine both your answers and your delivery. The more you practice, the more comfortable you will become in adapting to unexpected questions and presenting yourself with professionalism.

Ultimately, preparation and practice give you the confidence to walk into the interview, whether virtual or in person, knowing that you are ready to present the best version of yourself.

Common Questions and Best Answers

Residency interviews often follow a predictable structure, with a mix of general, behavioral, and IMG-specific questions.

Understanding the intention behind these questions and preparing structured, professional responses can make the difference between a strong interview and one that feels unfocused.

Below are some of the most common types of questions you can expect, along with strategies to craft answers that resonate with program directors.

One of the most frequently asked questions is, "Tell me about yourself." At first glance, this seems simple, but many applicants stumble by providing too much personal information or narrating their entire life story. The key is to keep your response professional, concise, and relevant to the role of a resident physician. For example, you might say: "I am a medical graduate from [Country] with strong clinical experience in internal medicine, complemented by U.S. rotations at [Hospitals]. My passion lies in primary care, and I am particularly interested in serving underserved populations." This kind of answer highlights your background, demonstrates U.S. experience, and introduces your career focus, all within a minute. It also provides a natural segue for the interviewer to ask follow-up questions about your rotations, research, or goals.

Another question you are almost certain to encounter is, "Why this specialty?" Program directors want to ensure that your choice of specialty is genuine and well thought out. This is where personal stories can have the most impact.

A meaningful patient encounter, a mentor who inspired you, or an experience that highlighted your skills can help illustrate why you are committed to a field.

For example, you may share how working with diabetic patients in your home country exposed you to the challenges of chronic disease management, sparking your interest in internal medicine.

The goal is to connect your specialty choice to your experiences, showing authenticity and passion rather than offering vague answers like “I like working with people.”

Equally important is the question, “Why this program?” Here, generic answers will quickly undermine your credibility. Program directors expect you to know their program’s strengths and be able to articulate how those strengths align with your goals.

Perhaps you were drawn to their patient demographics, such as the opportunity to work with immigrant populations. Maybe their structured mentorship program stands out, or their emphasis on research matches your academic interests.

Whatever the case, your answer should demonstrate that you have done your homework and can clearly articulate why you see yourself thriving there.

In addition to general questions, you should prepare for behavioral questions, which are designed to assess your interpersonal and problem-solving skills. A classic example is, “Tell me about a time you faced a conflict on a team.”

For this, the STAR method (Situation, Task, Action, Result) is invaluable.

You might describe a situation where team members disagreed on patient management, explain your role, highlight the actions you took to facilitate communication, and conclude with the resolution and what you learned.

Similarly, when asked, "Describe a situation where you had to adapt quickly," your answer should emphasize adaptability and resilience, qualities that programs expect, especially from IMGs who often face steep learning curves.

Finally, IMGs should be prepared for IMG-specific questions that probe motivation and cultural adaptability.

A common one is, "Why did you choose to practice in the U.S.?" Here, the best answers emphasize the positive aspects of U.S. training, such as exposure to diverse patient populations, structured residency programs, or a commitment to evidence-based medicine.

Avoid negative comparisons to your home country, as this may come across as dismissive or defensive.

Another frequently asked question is, "How will you handle cultural differences?" In answering, highlight your awareness and openness. For example: "I have trained in multiple healthcare systems, which taught me to adapt to new environments quickly and to respect diverse perspectives."

This not only shows humility but also reassures program directors that you can integrate smoothly into their teams.

By anticipating these common questions and preparing thoughtful, structured answers, IMGs can present themselves as confident, professional, and well aligned with the expectations of U.S. residency programs.

Red-Flag Questions

Programs may address:

- Gaps in training → Explain constructively (family responsibilities, exam preparation, research work).
- Low USMLE scores → Acknowledge briefly, then pivot to strengths (improvement, perseverance, U.S. experience).
- Visa status → Be honest but emphasize flexibility and long-term commitment.

Virtual vs. In-Person Interviews

The residency interview process has changed dramatically in the years following the COVID-19 pandemic.

Before 2020, nearly all interviews were conducted in person, requiring applicants to travel across the country to attend multiple sessions, often within a very short timeframe. However, the pandemic forced institutions to adapt quickly, and virtual interviews became the standard almost overnight. Even as restrictions have eased, many programs have continued with virtual formats, citing the benefits of accessibility and cost savings.

Some programs, however, are beginning to offer hybrid models, where candidates might attend initial rounds online and later be invited to visit the institution in person. For international medical graduates, this shift means it is now essential to be fully prepared for both virtual and in-person interviews, as the expectations and challenges of each format are different.

Virtual interviews offer clear advantages, particularly for IMGs who face significant logistical and financial hurdles when traveling. Costs associated with international flights, hotels, meals, and transportation can be prohibitive, and securing visas on short notice adds another layer of complexity. Virtual interviews remove these obstacles, allowing candidates to focus more on their preparation and performance rather than worrying about travel arrangements. Scheduling is also far simpler, with applicants able to interview with multiple programs across different states in a single week without leaving home.

Despite these benefits, virtual interviews present unique challenges.

One of the biggest drawbacks is the difficulty of building rapport. The subtleties of body language, casual conversations, and spontaneous interactions that occur in hallways or at social events are harder to replicate on a screen.

Candidates also miss out on the opportunity to experience the program's culture firsthand, walking through the hospital, observing residents at work, and getting a feel for the community where they might live and train.

To make the most of virtual interviews, attention to detail is critical. A professional background is non-negotiable. A neutral wall, proper lighting, and a quiet environment help keep the focus on you rather than distracting surroundings.

Good lighting, ideally natural light from a window or a ring light, ensures that your face is clearly visible and engaging. Technology checks are equally important. Testing your camera, microphone, and internet connection well in advance of the interview helps avoid awkward interruptions or technical failures. Even small things, like adjusting the height of your camera to eye level, can make a difference in how confident and polished you appear. It is also important to dress fully in professional attire, not just the visible upper half. This not only prevents embarrassing situations should you need to stand up, but also helps mentally prepare you to treat the interview with the same seriousness as an in-person meeting. Finally, maintaining eye contact is a subtle yet powerful skill. Instead of looking at the interviewer's image on the screen, try to focus on the camera itself. This gives the impression that you are speaking directly to the person, helping to create a stronger sense of connection.

While virtual formats dominate, some programs are beginning to reintroduce in-person interviews, particularly for final rounds or for specialties that place a high value on interpersonal interactions. For IMGs, these opportunities can be both exciting and daunting.

On the one hand, being physically present allows you to showcase qualities that are harder to convey virtually, such as warmth, confidence, and enthusiasm in casual settings. On the other hand, the logistical challenges of travel remain, and careful planning is essential.

If you are invited to an in-person interview, it is wise to arrange travel well in advance, especially if a visa is required. Arriving at least a day before the interview helps you recover from travel fatigue and ensures you are alert and prepared on the actual day.

One of the unique aspects of in-person interviews is the opportunity to participate in informal events, such as dinners or social gatherings with current residents. These occasions are not just social niceties, they are crucial parts of the evaluation process. Programs want to see how you interact in less formal settings, whether you ask thoughtful questions, and how well you connect with peers. Residents often provide feedback to program directors, so making a positive impression in these interactions can carry significant weight. Remember to remain professional even in casual settings, as every moment of the visit contributes to the overall impression you leave.

Ultimately, both virtual and in-person interviews have distinct advantages and challenges. Virtual interviews level the playing field by reducing costs and logistical barriers, but they require extra effort to convey warmth and connection through a screen. In-person interviews allow for richer interactions and a deeper understanding of the program environment but demand careful preparation and resources to execute smoothly.

For IMGs, being prepared for both formats ensures flexibility and confidence, no matter which type of interview a program uses. The key is to approach each format with professionalism, attention to detail, and a genuine interest in showcasing not only your qualifications but also your personality and adaptability.

Body Language, Professionalism, and Cultural Nuances

Body Language

Non-verbal cues often speak louder than words. U.S. interviewers value:

- Firm but not crushing handshakes (for in-person interviews).
- Sitting upright and avoiding crossed arms.
- Smiling and nodding to show engagement.
- Avoiding looking down or fidgeting excessively.

Professionalism

- Be punctual (log in 10 minutes early or arrive on site ahead of time).
- Address interviewers formally (Dr. Smith, not John).
- Thank them for their time at the end of the interview.

Cultural Nuances for IMGs

- Eye contact: In the U.S., steady eye contact shows confidence (but avoid staring aggressively).
- Direct answers: Avoid being vague; concise, structured responses are preferred.
- Humility with confidence: Show pride in your achievements without arrogance.

Following Up After Interviews

Thank-You Notes

Most programs appreciate a short thank-you email within 24 to 48 hours.

- Personalize it by mentioning something specific you discussed.
- Keep it professional: three to five sentences, with no spelling or grammatical errors.

Post-Interview Communication

Programs may send follow-up emails; respond promptly and professionally. Avoid excessive communication, which can appear desperate.

Ranking Strategy

After interviews, reflect on:

- Program culture and resident happiness.
- Fit with your career goals.

- Location, support systems, and long-term lifestyle.

Dealing with Rejection and Reapplication

Handling Rejection

Not every interview leads to a Match. Rejections are common and not necessarily a reflection of your ability.

- Normalize it: thousands of IMGs apply each year, and competition is fierce.
- Learn from feedback: if possible, ask mentors to review your performance.
- Stay resilient: use rejections as opportunities for growth.

Preparing for Reapplication

If unmatched, many IMGs successfully reapply. Strategies include:

- Gaining U.S. clinical experience (observerships, externships, research).
- Improving exam scores (Step 3 or subspecialty certifications).
- Strengthening application materials (updated personal statement, stronger letters of recommendation).
- Networking: attending conferences and connecting with program directors and residents.

Conclusion

The residency interview is the decisive stage in your IMG journey. More than test scores or documents, it reflects your character, adaptability, and readiness for U.S. medical training. With preparation, self-awareness, and resilience, you can navigate interviews confidently, whether virtual or in person, and present yourself as a future colleague, not just an applicant.

Remember that each interview is not only a chance for programs to assess you but also for you to evaluate them. Approach every interaction as a professional dialogue, and you will leave a lasting impression that strengthens your path to becoming a physician in the United States.

Chapter 9: Residency Life as an IMG

Residency is the bridge between medical school and independent practice. But for international medical graduates, it can feel like stepping into a completely new world. The transition goes far beyond medical knowledge, as it involves adapting to different systems, cultural expectations, and a demanding lifestyle.

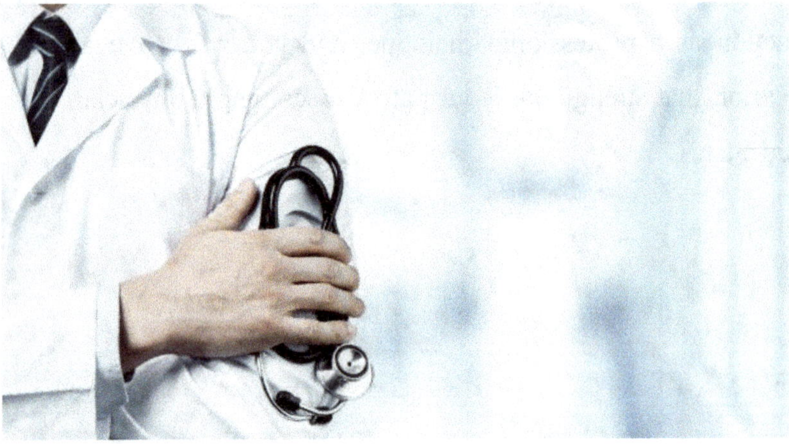

This chapter will explore what IMG residents can realistically expect during residency, how to adjust to the unique pressures of U.S. training, and what habits can help you not only survive but thrive.

Adjusting to Workload, Call Schedules, and Hierarchy

Managing Workload

Every resident entering a U.S. program quickly realizes that residency is not a 9-to-5 job. Typical duty hours are capped by the

Accreditation Council for Graduate Medical Education (ACGME) at 80 hours per week, averaged over four weeks. Still, many residents find themselves consistently near that limit. Shifts may last 12 to 28 hours, depending on the specialty, and call schedules can disrupt normal sleep patterns.

For IMGs, this can be an even sharper adjustment. Many international medical schools do not operate with the same level of continuity-of-care responsibility expected in U.S. residency. You may be the one writing orders, managing admissions at 2 a.m., and handling urgent phone calls from nurses overnight. Learning to function in a state of partial sleep deprivation, while keeping patient safety as the highest priority, is part of the rite of passage.

Understanding Hierarchy

U.S. residency programs are structured in a clear hierarchy. Interns (first-year residents) carry out much of the direct patient care under supervision. Senior residents supervise interns and make higher-level clinical decisions. Attendings (faculty physicians) oversee the team and ultimately bear legal responsibility for patient care. Beyond this, there are fellows in subspecialty programs, chief residents, and program leadership.

For IMGs who may come from cultures where hierarchy is either stricter or looser, adjusting to this balance can be tricky.

In the U.S., hierarchy exists, but open communication is encouraged. An intern can, and should, ask clarifying questions, raise safety concerns, or respectfully disagree if something seems unsafe.

Understanding when to speak up, how to document concerns, and how to escalate issues is part of learning the system.

Call Schedules and Shift Work

Residency is one of the most demanding stages of a medical career, and for international medical graduates, the adjustment can feel even more challenging.

One of the most difficult aspects to navigate is the unpredictable schedule and the intensity of shift work. Each specialty has its own rhythm and demands, requiring residents to be flexible and resilient in adapting to constantly changing hours.

Internal medicine and pediatrics residents, for example, often rotate through "night float" systems, where they work several consecutive nights before switching back to daytime duties. This can disrupt circadian rhythms and make it challenging to maintain a healthy routine.

Surgical residents, on the other hand, frequently start their days before dawn and end late in the evening, with shifts that can stretch over long hours and leave little time for personal rest.

For emergency medicine residents, schedules are even more erratic, involving frequent switches between day, evening, and overnight shifts.

This irregularity can take a physical and emotional toll, especially on IMGs who may not have a local family support system to lean on during stressful periods.

Tips for Adjusting to Workload and Hierarchy

Given this demanding schedule, developing strategies to manage workload becomes essential.

Sleep hygiene is a priority. Creating a dark, quiet environment for rest, even during the day, can help restore energy. Preparing quick, nutritious meals in advance ensures that eating does not become an afterthought. Some IMGs also benefit from maintaining small routines, such as short exercise sessions, prayer, or mindfulness practices, which bring a sense of grounding amid the chaos of residency life.

These habits may seem minor, but they provide much-needed stability in an otherwise unpredictable schedule.

Equally important is learning how to adjust to the hierarchical structure of residency programs.

Efficiency should be a focus from the very beginning. Developing a system for pre-rounding, learning to chart notes efficiently, and anticipating what senior residents or attending physicians will ask during rounds can help reduce stress and build confidence.

Respecting the chain of command is also crucial. Directing routine questions to senior residents before escalating to attendings not only demonstrates professionalism but also builds trust within the team.

Another key area for success lies in communication, especially with nurses. Nurses are often the first to notice subtle changes in a patient's condition, and building respectful, collaborative relationships with them can significantly improve patient care. Finally, IMGs must accept that mistakes and knowledge gaps are inevitable. No resident is perfect, and missteps will happen. What matters most is demonstrating the ability to learn quickly, adapt, and take responsibility. This attitude earns respect and fosters growth.

Residency schedules and hierarchies can feel overwhelming at first, but with deliberate strategies, humility, and resilience, IMGs can adapt and thrive in this demanding environment.

Cultural Dynamics with Patients, Nurses, and Fellow Residents

With Patients

Cultural differences can be one of the steepest learning curves for IMGs. Patients in the U.S. are often highly involved in their care decisions. They may question recommendations, request second opinions, or refuse treatments that you consider standard.

This is not a sign of disrespect, it reflects the U.S. healthcare emphasis on patient autonomy.

IMGs must learn to communicate medical information in plain English, avoid excessive jargon, and ensure patients understand risks and benefits. Empathy and listening skills often matter as much as clinical knowledge.

With Nurses

In many international systems, nurses are often seen as subordinates to physicians. In the U.S., however, nurses are autonomous professionals with significant authority. They may challenge orders if they believe something is unsafe, and they are often right.

Building respectful relationships with nurses is one of the fastest ways to succeed as a resident. Saying "thank you," listening to concerns, and collaborating go a long way.

With Fellow Residents

Your co-residents will be your closest allies during training. For IMGs, it can sometimes feel isolating if you are the only non-U.S. graduate in your class. However, sharing your story openly, showing humility, and supporting peers fosters genuine connections and bonds.

Remember that everyone struggles with long hours and stress, it is not just you.

Burnout, Mental Health, and Impostor Syndrome

Residency is often described as a trial by fire, and for many international medical graduates, the experience can feel even more overwhelming. Residency has one of the highest burnout rates among all professions, with studies showing that more than 40% of residents report symptoms of burnout at some point during training.

For IMGs, the risk is heightened by additional pressures such as visa uncertainties, cultural adaptation, and financial burdens tied to exams, relocation, and supporting families abroad. These stressors compound the already demanding workload, creating a perfect storm for mental health challenges if not carefully managed.

The sources of stress are numerous and often relentless. Sleep deprivation is nearly universal, with residents working long or irregular hours that disrupt natural rhythms. Constant performance evaluations can make residents feel as though they are always under a microscope, where one mistake may overshadow months of hard work.

The emotional toll of caring for critically ill patients, witnessing suffering, or dealing with patient deaths adds another layer of strain, particularly for those without strong local support networks. Isolation from loved ones in one's home country can deepen feelings of loneliness, while financial strain from licensing exams and the cost of living in the U.S. adds further pressure.

Adding to this burden is the experience of impostor syndrome. Many IMGs report feeling as though they do not truly belong or that they somehow "tricked" the system into accepting them into residency. Surrounded by peers who trained at prestigious U.S. medical schools, it is easy to fall into harsh self-comparisons.

Every small mistake may feel like confirmation of inadequacy, and the constant need to prove oneself can become exhausting. It is important to remember that every IMG in a residency program has earned their place. Selection committees choose candidates deliberately, recognizing resilience, adaptability, and diverse perspectives, qualities that enrich patient care and strengthen healthcare teams.

Coping with these challenges requires deliberate effort and a set of practical strategies.

Seeking peer support is one of the most powerful tools. Open conversations with co-residents often reveal shared struggles and normalize difficult emotions.

Many programs provide wellness resources such as counseling services, wellness workshops, or employee assistance programs, which can be invaluable when utilized.

On a personal level, mind-body practices, such as brief mindfulness exercises, breathing techniques, or short walks, can provide meaningful mental resets during demanding days.

Finally, seeking professional help should never be viewed as a weakness. Depression and anxiety are common during residency, and pursuing therapy, counseling, or medical care is an act of responsible self-care, not failure.

Ultimately, surviving residency as an IMG does not mean eliminating stress, it means learning to manage it effectively.

Recognizing burnout early, addressing impostor syndrome with self-compassion, and using available resources can transform residency from an experience of overwhelming strain into one of resilience and growth.

Visa Challenges During Residency

For international medical graduates, one of the biggest hurdles during residency is navigating the complexities of U.S. immigration law. While clinical work and adapting to a new healthcare system are already demanding, the added pressure of maintaining a valid visa status can weigh heavily.

Visa issues can influence not only where you match but also how smoothly your training progresses, your ability to visit family, and your long-term career options in the United States. Understanding the basics of visa types, the challenges you may face, and strategies to overcome them is essential to thriving as an IMG resident.

Visa Types

Most IMGs complete residency under one of two main visa categories. The first is the J-1 visa, also known as the Exchange Visitor Visa.

This visa is sponsored by the Educational Commission for Foreign Medical Graduates (ECFMG) and is the most common pathway for residency training. However, it comes with significant restrictions.

A J-1 visa typically requires you to return to your home country for at least two years after completing training, unless you are able to secure a waiver. Waivers often involve working in underserved areas for a period of three years, which can limit immediate career flexibility but also open opportunities in communities with a high need for physicians.

The second option is the H-1B visa, designated for specialty occupations. This visa is attractive because it allows for "dual intent," meaning you can apply for permanent residency while on H-1B status. It does not require the two-year return requirement associated with the J-1.

However, H-1B sponsorship is more difficult to obtain. Not every program is willing to go through the additional paperwork and costs required, and the process itself can be lengthy. For IMGs lucky enough to secure an H-1B, the pathway to long-term settlement in the U.S. is generally smoother, but competition for these positions is fierce.

Challenges Faced by IMGs

Visa challenges extend beyond simply securing sponsorship. One major issue is that not all residency programs are willing or able to sponsor visas, which narrows the field of potential matches for IMGs. Even after securing a visa, travel restrictions and delays in visa processing can make it difficult to return home for emergencies, holidays, or family events.

For those on J-1 visas, the two-year home residency requirement creates uncertainty and often forces graduates into specific waiver programs in underserved or rural areas, which may not align with personal or professional goals.

Another long-term challenge is the green card backlog. For IMGs from countries with high demand, such as India or China, the wait for permanent residency can stretch into many years. This uncertainty complicates career planning and adds another layer of stress during already demanding years of training.

Success Habits for Thriving as an IMG Resident

Residency in the United States is both a remarkable opportunity and one of the most demanding periods in an international medical graduate's career. The learning curve is steep, expectations are high, and the pressure to perform can feel relentless.

Yet, many IMGs not only survive but thrive by developing strong habits that support professional growth, personal well-being, and long-term goals. Building these habits early can make the difference between simply getting through residency and excelling in it.

Professional Habits

One of the most important professional habits for IMGs is punctuality. Arriving earlier than expected for rounds, conferences, or procedures sends a powerful message of reliability and respect for colleagues' time. In a system where efficiency is prized, arriving early also allows time to review charts, pre-round on patients, or prepare questions, helping you feel more confident and capable.

Another cornerstone of professionalism is thorough documentation. Writing clear and accurate notes is not just about meeting billing requirements. It demonstrates clinical reasoning and ensures continuity of care. Notes are often the first thing attendings, consultants, or even legal teams review if questions arise about a patient's course. Treating documentation as an extension of clinical judgment builds both credibility and legal protection.

Residency also marks the beginning of a career defined by lifelong learning. No matter how strong your foundation, medicine evolves daily. The most successful residents build the habit of reading around their cases each day. This does not require hours of study, just small, consistent efforts.Reviewing guidelines, reading a case report, or studying a management algorithm deepens understanding and builds confidence on rounds. Over time, this habit compounds, making you a stronger clinician and a more competitive candidate for fellowships or academic opportunities.

Personal Habits

Residency pushes the body as much as the mind, making sleep hygiene essential. With rotating shifts and overnight calls, rest is often fragmented.

Simple measures, such as blackout curtains, limiting caffeine late in the day, and reducing screen time before sleep, can maximize sleep quality. Even short naps before or after night shifts can provide meaningful recovery.

Nutrition is another area where habits make a major difference. It is easy to rely on hospital cafeteria food or vending machines, but these options rarely support sustained energy. Preparing simple meals in advance, carrying healthy snacks like nuts or fruit, and staying hydrated can stabilize mood and improve focus. Many residents find that modest meal preparation yields significant improvements in stamina during long shifts.

Exercise often feels like a luxury during residency, but even brief routines can be transformative. Ten to fifteen minutes of stretching, walking, or bodyweight exercises relieve tension, improve mood, and maintain physical resilience. Adopting the mindset that "something is better than nothing" helps avoid the all-or-nothing trap that derails healthy habits.

Social Habits

Residency can feel isolating, especially for IMGs who are far from home and family. Building a support network is therefore critical.

Friendships with co-residents, mentorship relationships with faculty, and involvement in cultural or religious organizations help prevent loneliness and provide balance outside of medicine.

Another sustaining habit is celebrating small wins. Residency is a marathon, and the years can blur together without moments of acknowledgment. Whether it is your first successful procedure, completing a challenging call rotation, or simply surviving your first night shift, recognizing milestones reinforces progress and motivation.

Maintaining connections with family abroad is equally important. Regular video calls, messages, or sharing small daily moments preserve emotional grounding. While physical distance may be unavoidable, strong relationships provide stability and support during difficult periods.

Long-Term Vision

Amid long hours, exams, and constant evaluations, it is easy to lose sight of the bigger picture. Reminding yourself that residency is temporary can serve as a stabilizing anchor. Whether your program lasts three years or seven, it is a stepping stone toward becoming a licensed, independent physician in the United States. Keeping this long-term vision in mind helps place daily struggles in perspective.

Residency is not only about enduring difficult schedules; it is about laying the foundation for the rest of your medical career. By developing strong professional, personal, and social habits, and keeping an eye on the goal, IMGs can thrive in residency and emerge as skilled physicians and resilient individuals prepared for the next chapter.

Conclusion

Residency as an IMG is both challenging and transformative. You will work harder than you ever imagined, face moments of self-doubt, and encounter cultural differences that test adaptability. Yet, you will also gain resilience, mastery, and the privilege of caring for patients in one of the most advanced healthcare systems in the world.

By preparing for workload and hierarchy, embracing cultural dynamics, protecting mental health, navigating visa hurdles, and building success habits, residency can become a powerful period of growth.

Every IMG's journey is unique, but one truth remains constant: your perspective, determination, and perseverance enrich the U.S. medical community in invaluable ways.

Chapter 10:

Beyond Residency - Fellowships and Practice

Completing residency as an international medical graduate is an extraordinary accomplishment. It represents years of preparation, adjustment, and resilience in navigating a complex U.S. system.

Yet, for many IMGs, residency is not the endpoint. The next phase, whether fellowship, independent practice, or alternative career pathways, brings new opportunities and challenges.

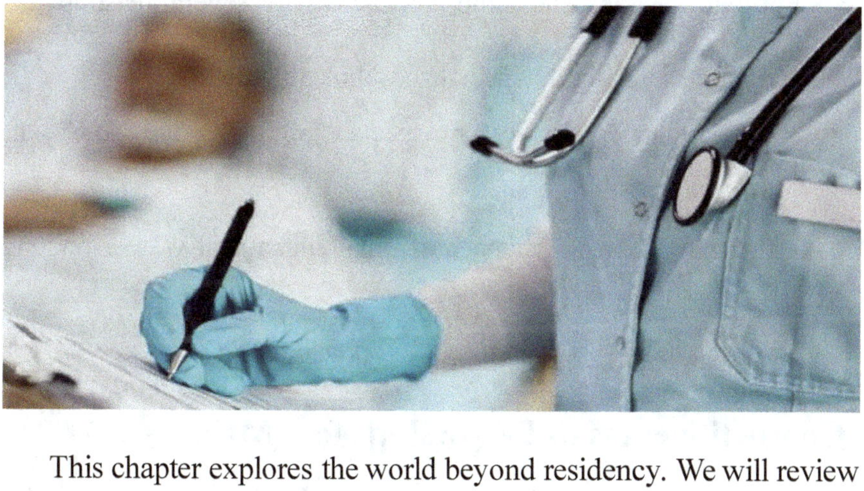

This chapter explores the world beyond residency. We will review fellowship opportunities available to IMGs, outline the requirements for independent practice, examine the visa and waiver hurdles many IMGs face, and highlight career paths that go beyond traditional clinical medicine.

The aim is to help you plan strategically so that your transition from trainee to physician-leader is smooth and successful.

Fellowship Opportunities for IMGs

A fellowship is additional subspecialty training pursued after residency. While residency provides broad exposure and prepares you for board certification in a core specialty (such as internal medicine, pediatrics, or surgery), fellowship allows you to refine expertise in a narrower field.

Examples include cardiology, gastroenterology, endocrinology, critical care, hematology/oncology, infectious diseases, and more.

For many IMGs, fellowship is attractive for several reasons:

- It provides highly specialized clinical skills.
- It enhances career prospects, both in the U.S. and internationally.
- It may improve chances of obtaining a visa waiver or long-term job stability.
- It can lead to academic or research-focused careers.

Competitiveness of Fellowships for IMGs

The fellowship application process for international medical graduates in the United States is primarily managed through the Electronic Residency Application Service (ERAS) and the National Resident Matching Program (NRMP) Specialties Matching Service. For IMGs, understanding the relative competitiveness of fellowships is crucial in setting realistic expectations and strategically planning career steps. Competitiveness varies widely depending on the specialty, the applicant pool, and the specific program.

Highly competitive fellowships, such as cardiology, gastroenterology, dermatology, and surgical subspecialties, are among the most difficult to secure. These specialties attract a large number of applicants, both U.S. graduates and IMGs, which raises the bar significantly.

Successful IMG applicants usually bring strong U.S.-based research experience, high scores on in-service and board examinations, and compelling letters of recommendation from well-respected faculty.

In these fields, having a robust research portfolio, ideally with publications in high-impact journals, can often make the difference.

Moderately competitive specialties include endocrinology, nephrology, hematology/oncology, and pulmonary and critical care. These fields remain highly respected and rewarding but tend to have slightly more openings compared to the applicant pool. For IMGs, this means there is still a substantial challenge, but strong clinical performance and mentorship can provide a significant edge. Many applicants in these specialties succeed by demonstrating consistent interest in the field through electives, research, and conference participation.

More IMG-friendly fellowships include infectious diseases, geriatrics, and palliative care. These specialties are critical for the healthcare system but often receive fewer applications compared to highly competitive fields. IMGs with solid residency performance, a reliable work ethic, and demonstrated passion for patient-centered care have a greater chance of matching in these programs. While research and networking remain valuable, strong emphasis is placed on clinical skills, professionalism, and a commitment to serving underserved populations.

Ultimately, the same strategies that helped IMGs succeed in matching into residency apply here: showcasing clinical excellence, building mentorship relationships, and aligning personal goals with the mission and needs of the fellowship program.

Building a Fellowship-Ready Profile

To maximize the chances of securing a fellowship, IMGs need to begin preparing early in residency. Creating a strong fellowship-ready profile involves a multifaceted approach:

Research: A solid research foundation is essential for competitive specialties but valuable across all fields. Publications, abstracts, and posters in your chosen specialty help establish credibility and showcase intellectual curiosity. Even case reports or quality improvement projects can add depth to your application.

The key is consistency, steady contributions during residency reflect both interest and initiative.

Mentorship: One of the most powerful assets an IMG can have is a strong mentor. Senior faculty who are well connected in your subspecialty can provide not only guidance but also advocacy when fellowship directors seek references. Building these relationships takes effort, showing dedication on rounds, volunteering for academic projects, and maintaining professionalism are effective ways to foster mentorship connections.

Performance during residency: Fellowship directors often seek evaluations from program directors and senior faculty. Excelling in day-to-day clinical duties, demonstrating teamwork, and taking ownership of patient care can leave lasting impressions. In many cases, strong clinical evaluations can outweigh modest research output.

Networking: Finally, networking plays a critical role. Attending national conferences, such as those hosted by the American College of Cardiology or the American Society of Clinical Oncology, allows IMGs to meet leaders in the field, explore fellowship opportunities, and demonstrate enthusiasm. Active engagement, asking thoughtful questions, presenting research, and participating in poster sessions, can significantly enhance visibility.

By focusing on these areas, IMGs can position themselves as well-rounded candidates who bring both clinical strength and academic potential. Whether aiming for a highly competitive subspecialty or a more IMG-friendly field, the consistent thread remains the same: preparation, persistence, and professionalism.

Alternative Fellowship Pathways

Some IMGs pursue non-ACGME fellowships in areas such as research, hospital medicine, or global health. These may not lead to board certification but can enhance expertise and career development. Others consider one-year "pre-fellowship" research positions if they do not match immediately. These can act as stepping stones, though they may delay independent practice.

Licensing Requirements for Independent Practice

State Medical Licensure

Finishing residency or fellowship does not automatically grant the ability to practice independently. Each U.S. state has its own medical board that sets requirements for full licensure. While details differ, common requirements include:

- Graduation from a recognized medical school.
- Completion of at least one to three years of accredited residency training in the U.S. (some states require full residency completion for IMGs).
- Passing all required exams (USMLE Step 1, Step 2 CK, and Step 3).
- Background checks, fingerprinting, and verification of credentials.

USMLE Step 3 and Licensure

For IMGs, Step 3 is critical. While Step 1 and Step 2 CK allow entry into residency, Step 3 is required for full medical licensure. Many states require IMGs to complete Step 3 before granting a license, even after residency completion.

Interstate Medical Licensure Compact (IMLC)

As of 2025, more than 35 states participate in the Interstate Medical Licensure Compact, which streamlines the process of applying for multiple state licenses. If you plan to work in telemedicine or across multiple states, this can be an advantage. However, eligibility requires that your primary license be in a participating state and that you meet specific criteria, such as board certification.

Board Certification

Beyond licensure, many employers and hospitals require board certification in your specialty. This involves passing written and, in some cases, oral board examinations administered by specialty-specific boards under the American Board of Medical Specialties (ABMS) or equivalent organizations. Fellowship graduates may then sit for subspecialty boards, such as cardiology after internal medicine.

Navigating J-1 Waiver Programs for Underserved Areas

For many international medical graduates, the J-1 visa is the most common route for training in U.S. residency and fellowship programs. While it opens the door to advanced training, the J-1 visa also comes with strict conditions, including the two-year home-country return rule.

Fortunately, waiver programs exist to help IMGs continue their medical careers in the United States while addressing critical physician shortages in underserved communities. Understanding these waiver programs, their requirements, and their challenges is essential for planning a successful career path.

The J-1 Visa and Its Two-Year Rule

Most IMGs enter U.S. graduate medical education on a J-1 visa sponsored by the Educational Commission for Foreign Medical Graduates (ECFMG).

Under immigration law, once training is completed, physicians are required to return to their home country for a period of two years before applying for certain immigration benefits, such as permanent residency or an H-1B visa. This requirement can be a major roadblock for IMGs who wish to remain in the United States to practice medicine.

To bypass this restriction, physicians can obtain a J-1 waiver by committing to serve in areas with significant healthcare shortages. Typically, this involves working for at least three years in a medically underserved or rural region.

While this path is demanding, it allows IMGs to gain valuable work experience, build careers in the U.S., and contribute meaningfully to communities with limited access to care.

The Conrad 30 Waiver Program

The most widely known and utilized waiver option is the Conrad 30 Waiver Program. Under this program, each U.S. state can sponsor up to 30 J-1 physicians per year to work in underserved areas. The Conrad 30 program was created to balance the need for qualified physicians with the shortage of medical professionals in rural and inner-city communities.

Competition for Conrad 30 slots varies considerably from state to state. In some states with large IMG populations and urban centers, the slots fill up quickly, sometimes within days of applications opening. In other states, especially those with more rural settings, slots may remain unfilled for months, giving applicants more flexibility.

Key considerations for IMGs include:

- **Employment requirements:** You must secure a full-time job offer from an eligible employer located in a Health Professional Shortage Area (HPSA) or Medically Underserved Area (MUA).
- **Application timing:** States typically open applications once a year, and timing is critical. Submitting early can significantly improve your chances.

- **Employer support:** Many sponsoring employers provide immigration attorney assistance to help with paperwork, making the process smoother.

For IMGs, the Conrad 30 program is often the first step toward building long-term stability in the U.S. medical system.

Other Waiver Options

While the Conrad 30 program is the most common path, there are other waiver opportunities available for IMGs:

- **Federal programs:** Certain regional organizations, such as the Appalachian Regional Commission (ARC) and the Delta Regional Authority (DRA), offer J-1 waivers for physicians willing to practice in their designated service areas. These programs expand the pool of opportunities beyond the state-based Conrad 30 limit.
- **VA facilities:** The U.S. Department of Veterans Affairs (VA) can sponsor physicians for J-1 waivers without being restricted by the 30-per-state cap. For IMGs interested in serving veterans, this can be an excellent option.
- **Hardship waivers:** In rare cases, waivers may be granted if returning to the home country would cause undue hardship to a U.S. citizen spouse or child, or if the physician would face persecution. These are less common but remain an important safeguard.

Challenges for IMGs

While J-1 waiver programs open the door to long-term practice in the U.S., they also come with challenges. Waiver positions are often located in rural towns or resource-limited healthcare settings where patient needs are high, but resources and support staff may be limited. For IMGs, this can require rapid adaptation, self-reliance, and resilience.

Yet, these challenges also bring unique rewards. Working in underserved areas allows physicians to gain independence early in their careers, take on leadership responsibilities, and make a visible impact on communities in need.

Many physicians later reflect on these years as formative, not only for their clinical skills but also for their personal growth. After fulfilling the three-year commitment, IMGs often transition to other roles, pursue fellowships, or move into urban practices with a stronger professional foundation.

Navigating J-1 waiver programs can seem daunting at first, but for IMGs, they represent both an opportunity and a bridge to long-term practice in the United States. By understanding the available options, from the widely used Conrad 30 program to federal and hardship waivers, physicians can align their career goals with pathways that meet immigration requirements while serving vital healthcare needs across the country.

Transitioning from Training to Attending Roles

Shifting Mindset

Residency and fellowship are supervised learning environments. As an attending physician, you become the final authority. This shift requires confidence, decisiveness, and the ability to mentor others. Many IMGs initially struggle with this responsibility, especially if they come from hierarchical systems where seniority strictly dictates decision-making.

Leadership Responsibilities

Attending physicians supervise residents, manage teams, and often balance clinical, administrative, and teaching duties. Skills in conflict resolution, delegation, and communication become as important as clinical knowledge.

Financial Transition

The jump from resident salary to attending salary is often dramatic. This allows IMGs to pay down educational debt, send money home, or invest in long-term goals. However, financial literacy is crucial. Physicians who do not plan for taxes, retirement savings, or loan repayment may quickly feel overwhelmed.

Career Options: Academia, Research, Private Practice, Public Health

Once visa concerns are addressed and board certification is secured, IMGs can explore a broad range of career paths in the U.S.

healthcare system. Each pathway comes with unique rewards, challenges, and long-term opportunities.

Academia

For IMGs who enjoy teaching, mentorship, and research, academic medicine offers a fulfilling career. Academic physicians balance several roles: caring for patients, educating medical students and residents, and engaging in scholarly activities such as research and publications.

Faculty positions also open doors to leadership roles, from directing residency programs to shaping curricula or chairing departments.

Success in academia often hinges on maintaining a strong scholarly record. Publishing in peer-reviewed journals, securing grant funding, and presenting at national conferences are crucial for promotion. IMGs who demonstrated research productivity during residency or fellowship may have a smoother transition. Additionally, assuming formal mentorship roles can enhance both professional reputation and institutional value. While academic salaries may be lower than those in private practice, the intellectual environment and influence on the next generation of physicians can be highly rewarding.

Research Careers

Some IMGs pursue careers in full-time research, either as physician-scientists or clinical researchers. Opportunities exist in universities, dedicated research institutes, hospitals, and the pharmaceutical industry.

Areas of focus may include basic science, translational medicine, or clinical trials.

A successful research career typically requires fellowship training with substantial time devoted to projects, grants, and publications. Funding remains competitive, and IMGs may need strong mentorship from established investigators to navigate the U.S. research ecosystem.

For those passionate about discovery, research careers allow physicians to contribute to advancements that impact patient care globally, even beyond direct clinical practice.

Private Practice

Private practice remains a traditional and attractive career route, especially for IMGs seeking greater autonomy. Physicians may join an established group practice or, with experience, open their own. Private practice often offers higher earning potential and more control over work schedules compared to academic or hospital-employed roles.

However, success in private practice requires more than clinical expertise. Physicians must navigate business management, billing systems, and health insurance policies.

Understanding the U.S. healthcare market is essential, as physicians must balance patient care with financial sustainability. For entrepreneurial IMGs, private practice provides independence and the opportunity to build long-term patient relationships.

Public Health and Policy

With global perspectives and cross-cultural experience, IMGs are well positioned to contribute to public health, epidemiology, and health policy. Many pursue advanced degrees, such as an MPH (Master of Public Health), to complement clinical training. Careers may involve work with government agencies like the Centers for Disease Control and Prevention (CDC), international organizations such as the World Health Organization (WHO), or non-governmental organizations (NGOs).

Public health roles emphasize population-level interventions, disease prevention, and health equity. IMGs with firsthand experience in international healthcare systems bring valuable insight into addressing disparities in the U.S. and globally.

Industry Roles

The healthcare industry increasingly recruits physicians into non-clinical roles, particularly within pharmaceutical and biotechnology companies. Positions in medical affairs, clinical development, and regulatory strategy allow IMGs to apply their medical expertise without direct patient care.

These roles may involve overseeing clinical trials, ensuring regulatory compliance, or serving as liaisons between research teams and healthcare providers.

For IMGs with strong research backgrounds, communication skills, or an interest in innovation, industry careers offer diverse opportunities, competitive compensation, and exposure to cutting-edge science.

Conclusion

Beyond residency, IMGs face both daunting challenges and exciting opportunities. Fellowships open doors to specialized expertise, licensure provides the foundation for independent practice, waiver programs create pathways for long-term careers in the U.S., and diverse career tracks allow IMGs to align professional life with personal values.

The transition from trainee to attending is more than a career milestone, it is the realization of years of perseverance and adaptation. Whether you choose clinical medicine, academia, research, or public health, your journey as an IMG brings unique strengths to American healthcare.

By staying informed, cultivating mentorship, and planning strategically, you can transform the hurdles of residency into the foundation for a rewarding and impactful future.

Chapter 11: Transitioning from Practicing Physician Abroad to U.S. Trainee

For many international medical graduates, the journey to a U.S. residency involves not only mastering exams and applications but also navigating one of the most profound professional adjustments of their lives: moving from being a practicing physician in their home country to starting again as a supervised trainee in the United States. This chapter is designed specifically for physicians who have already completed their MD, practiced medicine independently, and now face the challenge of re-entering the medical hierarchy for residency at a junior level.

This transition can feel humbling, frustrating, and sometimes disorienting, but it also opens the door to new growth, opportunities, and integration into one of the world's most advanced healthcare systems.

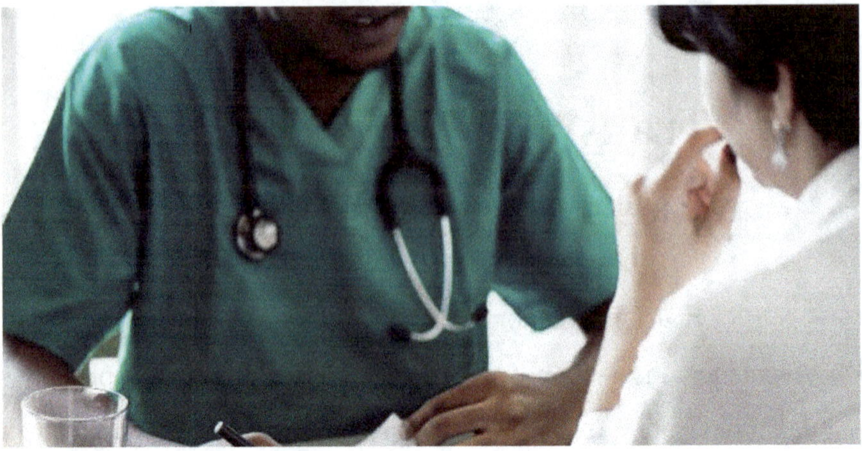

Understanding the emotional, professional, and cultural aspects of this shift will help you adapt more smoothly and thrive as a resident physician in the U.S.

The Emotional and Professional Shift: From Independent Practice to Supervised Training

One of the most difficult transitions for experienced international physicians is accepting the new identity of a "trainee."

In many countries, doctors who have completed an MD or MBBS and subsequent internship move quickly into independent practice. By the time they consider training abroad, many have built successful careers: they see patients daily, perform procedures, supervise junior doctors, and enjoy respect in their communities.

Arriving in the U.S. for residency can feel like stepping backward. You may suddenly find yourself reporting to younger colleagues, asking permission before making clinical decisions, and being evaluated at every step. Instead of being the authority figure, you are once again the learner.

This change often triggers mixed emotions:

- **Loss of Status:** Physicians accustomed to being addressed as "Doctor" by patients and peers may struggle with the reduced autonomy of residency. In some institutions, attendings and staff may not immediately recognize your prior qualifications.
- **Self-Doubt:** You may question whether all your years of training and practice abroad are valued in the U.S. healthcare system.
- **Identity Conflict:** Many IMGs describe feeling "caught between two worlds", a respected professional in their home country, yet a novice in the United States.
- **Excitement and Renewal:** On the positive side, many physicians also feel invigorated by the opportunity to learn new techniques, access advanced technology, and participate in world-class medical education.

It is important to recognize that these feelings are normal. Nearly every IMG with prior practice experience undergoes this emotional recalibration. What matters is how you process the change and position yourself to succeed.

Reframing Expectations: Hierarchy, Decision-Making, and Scope of Practice

1. Understanding Hierarchy in U.S. Residency

The American residency system is structured and hierarchical, with clear lines of supervision:

- **Intern (PGY-1):** Responsible for day-to-day patient care, order entry, initial assessments, and routine communication.
- **Resident (PGY-2 and PGY-3):** Greater responsibility for decision-making, supervision of interns and medical students, and coordination of care.
- **Chief Resident (PGY-3 or PGY-4, depending on specialty):** Leadership, scheduling, and liaison between faculty and residents.
- **Fellow (post-residency):** Subspecialty training with significant autonomy.
- **Attending Physician:** Final responsibility for patient care, supervision of all trainees, teaching, and independent practice.

Even if you were the equivalent of an attending abroad, you will need to operate within this structure. Decisions, even seemingly routine ones, may require attending approval. Understanding this hierarchy prevents frustration and helps you integrate into team dynamics.

2. Decision-Making Dynamics

In many healthcare systems abroad, physicians, especially in private practice, enjoy wide autonomy. In the U.S., decision-making is more collaborative and involves multiple stakeholders: nurses, pharmacists, social workers, and case managers. Residents are expected to consult with attendings and often require explicit approval before initiating treatment plans.

This does not diminish your skills; instead, it reflects the medico-legal environment and the culture of interprofessional collaboration in U.S. hospitals.

3. Scope of Practice

Residency in the U.S. is both broader and narrower than independent practice abroad. As a resident, you will:

- Perform procedures and manage patients, but only within the scope defined by your program and attending supervision.
- Participate in rotations across subspecialties, sometimes repeating areas in which you already have significant expertise.
- Gain exposure to U.S.-specific healthcare issues such as electronic health record (EHR) systems, insurance-driven care, and regulatory compliance (HIPAA, billing, coding).

Reframing residency not as a "step backward," but as an opportunity to expand your medical toolbox, will help you make the most of the experience.

Balancing Professional Pride with Humility in a New System

Finding the right balance between acknowledging your prior experience and embracing humility as a learner is essential. Too much emphasis on your background may come across as arrogance, while minimizing your expertise entirely may prevent you from leveraging strengths that make you an asset to your program.

Practical Tips for Balancing Pride and Humility:

1. **Acknowledge Your Experience Thoughtfully:** Share your background when it adds value, for example, if you have managed certain conditions frequently or performed specific procedures extensively. Frame it as a resource for the team rather than a challenge to authority.

2. **Respect U.S. Protocols:** Even if you know alternative approaches that worked abroad, defer to U.S. guidelines unless invited to discuss them. Showing adaptability signals professionalism.

3. **Adopt a Growth Mindset:** Approach residency as an advanced fellowship in "U.S. medicine." Even if you repeat familiar rotations, view them as opportunities to understand system-based practice, not just clinical skills.

4. **Seek Feedback Proactively:** Ask attendings and senior residents for input on how you can improve. This demonstrates humility and eagerness to learn.
5. **Practice Cultural Humility:** Remember that patients come from diverse backgrounds, and cultural competence is as important as medical expertise in the U.S.

The most successful IMGs project confidence without overstepping, drawing on their prior expertise to enrich the team while respecting the training structure.

Case Studies: Successful Transitions

Case Study 1: Dr. R from India Dr. R completed her MBBS and MD in Internal Medicine in India, where she practiced for six years. Accustomed to being the sole decision-maker in her private clinic, she initially struggled with the residency hierarchy in the U.S. During her PGY-1 year in Internal Medicine, she felt frustrated having to "check every order" with her attending. Over time, she reframed the experience as an opportunity to learn the U.S. system's emphasis on teamwork. By her PGY-2 year, she became a valued mentor to younger IMGs, helping them adapt emotionally. Today, she is a hospitalist and credits her success to embracing humility early in training.

Case Study 2: Dr. O from Nigeria Dr. O had been a general surgeon in Nigeria for nearly a decade before moving to the U.S. for family reasons. He matched into a General Surgery residency but found it difficult to accept being supervised by attendings younger than himself. Instead of resisting, he focused on mastering laparoscopic techniques and advanced imaging that were less available in Nigeria.

His positive attitude made him a role model in his program. After residency, he pursued a fellowship and now combines U.S. and African surgical practices in global health initiatives.

Case Study 3: Dr. M from Mexico Dr. M was a pediatrician in Mexico with 12 years of experience. During her pediatrics residency in the U.S., she initially felt disheartened when asked to “prove” her competence in procedures she had performed countless times.

She approached the situation by mentoring medical students and sharing insights about managing limited-resource settings.

Her program valued her unique perspective, and she was later appointed Chief Resident. Her advice to other IMGs: “See residency not as repeating what you already know, but as gaining a second education in a new culture.”

Strategies for Maintaining Confidence While Adapting to a Junior Role

Maintaining confidence while adjusting to a junior role is one of the greatest challenges for experienced international physicians. The following strategies can help:

1. Reframe the Narrative

Instead of thinking, "I am starting over," think, "I am upgrading my skill set for a new system." Residency becomes less about repeating training and more about adaptation and enhancement.

2. Celebrate Transferable Skills

Even if you are in a supervised role, you bring valuable assets: diagnostic reasoning, bedside manner, resilience under pressure, and years of patient care experience. Recognize these as strengths that make you stand out.

3. Build Peer Support

Seek out other IMGs who share similar backgrounds. IMG support groups, WhatsApp communities, or institutional mentorship programs can provide emotional solidarity and practical advice.

4. Maintain Professional Identity

Keep in touch with professional networks in your home country. Publishing research, attending international conferences, or participating in global health projects can reinforce your sense of identity as a physician, not "just a resident."

5. Practice Self-Care

Residency is demanding, and stress is magnified when combined with cultural adjustment. Prioritize sleep, nutrition, exercise, and mental health. Many programs now provide wellness resources; do not hesitate to use them.

6. Use Your Unique Perspective

Your international background gives you a broader lens. Share insights on tropical diseases, limited-resource care, or patient communication styles from your home country. This enriches your residency program and reminds you of your value.

7. Focus on Long-Term Goals

Residency is temporary. Keep your eyes on the bigger picture: becoming a board-certified U.S. physician, advancing your career, and contributing to global health. This perspective helps you endure the temporary challenges of hierarchy.

Conclusion

Transitioning from a practicing physician abroad to a resident in the U.S. is one of the most profound shifts in the IMG journey. It requires emotional resilience, humility, and adaptability. While it can feel like a step backward, in reality, it is a strategic step forward, an investment in building a career that blends international experience with U.S. medical training.

By reframing expectations, balancing pride with humility, learning from others who have made the transition, and maintaining confidence in your abilities, you can not only survive but thrive in this journey.

Remember that you bring invaluable experience, perspective, and resilience to your residency program. Your path may look different from that of your U.S.-trained peers, but it is no less valid. In many ways, it enriches the very fabric of American medicine.

Chapter 12: Specialty Choice for Experienced Physicians

For international medical graduates who have already completed an MD and practiced medicine abroad, one of the most consequential decisions in pursuing a U.S. residency is choosing a specialty.

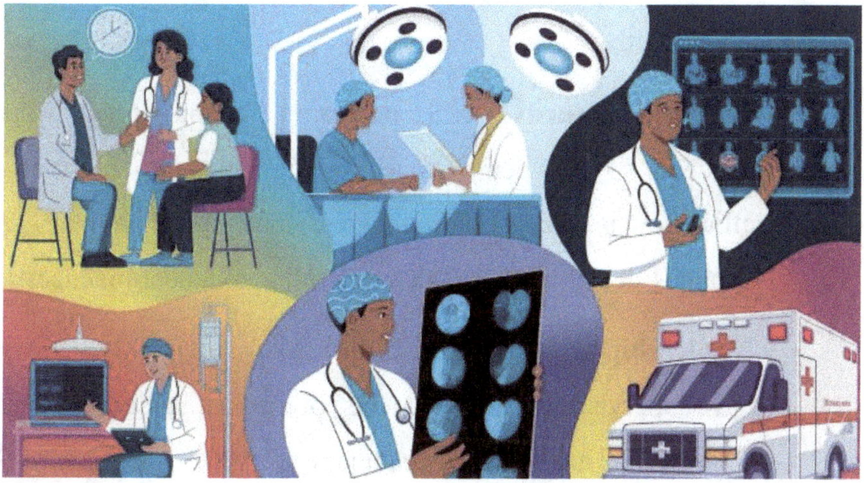

Unlike fresh graduates, you bring years of training, clinical practice, and often leadership experience. While this background can strengthen your application, it also raises unique challenges: How do you decide whether to repeat the same specialty you practiced at home or pivot to a different field? Which specialties are most receptive to internationally trained doctors? And how can you leverage your experience without appearing "overqualified"?

This chapter will guide you through the specialty decision-making process, highlight competitive realities, and provide strategies to align your prior expertise with U.S. residency opportunities.

How Prior Experience Shapes Residency Competitiveness

1. Advantages of Prior Practice Experience

Your years as a practicing physician can be a tremendous asset if positioned correctly:

- **Clinical Maturity:** U.S. program directors often value residents who demonstrate strong clinical reasoning, efficiency in patient care, and resilience under pressure, all qualities developed through years of independent practice.
- **Leadership and Teaching Skills:** Many experienced IMGs have supervised interns, residents, or medical students abroad. This background signals readiness to mentor peers in U.S. programs.
- **Research and Publications:** Physicians from academic hospitals abroad may already have publications, bolstering their residency competitiveness.
- **Adaptability to Stress:** Long hours, high patient volumes, and resource-limited settings abroad foster resilience, a trait residency directors prize.

2. Potential Challenges

However, prior practice can also create hurdles:

- **Perception of Overqualification:** Some program directors may wonder whether an experienced physician will adapt well to supervision by younger attendings.
- **Time Since Graduation (TSG):** Programs often screen applicants based on recency of graduation. A doctor who finished medical school 10 to 15 years ago may face automatic filters, regardless of practice history.
- **Mismatch Between Skills and Role:** If you were a surgeon abroad, being asked to relearn basics under close oversight may feel frustrating and create tension.
- **Licensure Gaps:** Clinical skills honed abroad may not always align with U.S. standards, such as electronic health record use, documentation practices, and malpractice-driven care.

The key is to emphasize the advantages while addressing potential concerns proactively in your application and interviews.

Choosing Between Repeating the Same Specialty vs. Pivoting to a New One

Repeating the Same Specialty

Many IMGs naturally want to continue in the specialty they trained for and practiced abroad. If you were a pediatrician, surgeon, or psychiatrist, the thought of starting over in another field may feel disorienting.

Staying in your field allows you to:

- Build on existing expertise
- Showcase depth of clinical experience
- Position yourself as a future leader who bridges international and U.S. practices

Example: A cardiologist from India applying for Internal Medicine residency with a plan to subspecialize in Cardiology in the U.S. highlights their years of echocardiography and interventional experience to strengthen their application.

Potential Challenge: Highly competitive specialties (e.g., dermatology, neurosurgery) may not be realistic, even for seasoned physicians. Programs often prioritize U.S. graduates for these fields.

Pivoting to a New Specialty

Some IMGs choose to change direction for pragmatic or personal reasons:

- **Competitiveness:** If your specialty is extremely competitive in the U.S., pivoting increases your match chances.
- **Lifestyle:** Many physicians reevaluate lifestyle priorities when relocating; some pivot from surgery to family medicine or psychiatry to achieve work–life balance.

- **Interest in New Opportunities:** U.S. residency offers exposure to fields not widely available in some countries, such as palliative care, hospitalist medicine, or clinical informatics.

Example: A surgeon from Nigeria who realized general surgery was highly competitive pivoted to Family Medicine, matched successfully, and later integrated minor surgical procedures into primary care practice.

Key Consideration: Identity and Long-Term Goals

Ask yourself: *Do I see myself repeating years of training in the same specialty, or am I ready to redefine my professional identity?* There is no "one size fits all" answer. The right choice depends on your competitiveness, family needs, and career vision.

Specialties That Value Prior Practice Experience

Certain specialties are consistently more welcoming to IMGs, particularly those with prior clinical backgrounds.

1. Internal Medicine (IM)

- **Why It's IMG-Friendly:** Internal Medicine consistently ranks as one of the largest specialties in the Match, with thousands of positions available annually. IMGs historically account for a significant proportion of these spots.
- **Value of Prior Experience:** If you practiced as a general physician, internist, or hospitalist abroad, your experience

directly aligns. Prior patient volume and familiarity with chronic disease management are strong assets.

- **Career Pathways:** Hospitalist medicine, cardiology, gastroenterology, and infectious disease are natural extensions for IMGs with prior IM backgrounds.

2. Family Medicine (FM)

- **Why It's IMG-Friendly:** With a strong focus on primary care and underserved communities, FM programs often welcome IMGs, particularly those willing to work in rural or shortage areas.
- **Value of Prior Experience:** Physicians who worked in general practice or community health abroad are especially well prepared. Experience in women's health, pediatrics, and preventive care is highly valued.
- **Career Pathways:** Outpatient practice, rural health, global health, and academic roles are common.

3. Psychiatry

- **Why It's IMG-Friendly:** Psychiatry has grown more competitive in recent years, but programs still value mature, diverse candidates. The global rise in mental health awareness has expanded residency positions.
- **Value of Prior Experience:** International physicians who managed mental health conditions in resource-limited settings bring unique perspectives. Cultural competence is a significant asset in psychiatry.

- **Career Pathways:** Community psychiatry, child and adolescent psychiatry, and addiction medicine offer further specialization.

4. Pediatrics

- **Why It's Moderately IMG-Friendly:** Pediatrics programs often welcome IMGs, particularly those who practiced abroad in high-volume pediatric settings.
- **Value of Prior Experience:** Pediatricians from Latin America or Asia often bring broad experience across outpatient and inpatient pediatrics, which can distinguish them in the Match.

5. Pathology

- **Why It's IMG-Friendly:** Pathology programs historically have a higher percentage of IMGs.
- **Value of Prior Experience:** If you practiced pathology abroad, your research and diagnostic skills may translate well, though additional U.S.-based exposure is often necessary.

Specialties Where Barriers Remain Higher Despite Experience

While prior practice is valuable, some specialties remain disproportionately difficult for IMGs to enter, regardless of their background.

1. Dermatology

- **Barrier:** Extremely competitive with limited residency positions. Programs prioritize U.S. graduates with strong research backgrounds.
- **Reality for IMGs:** Even experienced dermatologists abroad often pivot to Internal Medicine or Family Medicine and later pursue aesthetic medicine or dermatology-related fellowships outside the Match.

2. Orthopedic Surgery

- **Barrier:** High demand, rigorous procedural training, and fewer residency slots.
- **Reality for IMGs:** Prior surgical experience rarely outweighs the bias toward U.S. graduates. Only a small handful of IMGs match each year.

3. Neurosurgery

- **Barrier:** Long training duration, high liability, and limited residency positions.
- **Reality for IMGs:** Matching is rare; many foreign-trained neurosurgeons pivot to research, neurocritical care, or neurology.

4. Plastic Surgery

- **Barrier:** Among the most competitive specialties, with significant emphasis on research productivity.

- **Reality for IMGs:** Foreign-trained plastic surgeons often find more opportunities in non-ACGME fellowships or aesthetic practices after completing a different residency.

5. Radiation Oncology and Ophthalmology

- **Barrier:** Both are small fields with very few residency slots. U.S. graduates overwhelmingly dominate the Match.

Bottom Line: If you are deeply committed to one of these fields, you must demonstrate exceptional research, strong U.S. clinical experience, and mentorship from U.S. faculty. Otherwise, it may be more strategic to pivot.

Tailoring Applications to Highlight International Expertise While Fitting U.S. Expectations

Your application must strike a delicate balance: showcasing your international accomplishments while fitting the mold of a U.S. residency applicant.

1. Personal Statement

- Highlight how your international experience shaped your clinical perspective.
- Frame prior practice as preparation for adapting quickly to U.S. training.
- Emphasize humility and eagerness to learn U.S.-specific systems.

Example: "While managing hundreds of patients in my rural clinic in India taught me resilience and efficiency, I now seek structured residency training to integrate these skills with evidence-based medicine practiced in the U.S."

2. Curriculum Vitae (CV)

- Reframe titles: Instead of *"Consultant Cardiologist,"* use *"Attending Physician (equivalent to U.S. attending)"* with a brief explanation.
- Focus on achievements relevant to U.S. residency: patient care, procedures, teaching, and research.
- Limit detail on administrative or private-practice roles that may appear less relevant.

3. Letters of Recommendation (LORs)

- Strong U.S.-based LORs are essential. Even if you were a senior physician abroad, programs rely heavily on U.S. faculty endorsements.
- International letters can supplement but should not replace U.S. references.

4. ERAS Application

- Be transparent about time since graduation. Address gaps with meaningful activities such as research, observerships, or volunteering.

- Emphasize continuity of medical engagement, even if you were in non-clinical roles.

5. Interview Preparation

- Be ready to explain why you are pursuing residency in the U.S. after practicing abroad.
- Practice responses to "Why this specialty?" that balance passion with pragmatism.
- Demonstrate openness to supervision and enthusiasm for team-based learning.

Conclusion

Choosing a specialty as an experienced physician entering the U.S. residency system is both a professional and personal crossroads. Your prior experience is a powerful asset, but it must be presented in a way that resonates with U.S. program directors and acknowledges the realities of the Match.

For some, repeating the same specialty provides continuity and an opportunity to deepen expertise. For others, pivoting to more IMG-friendly specialties opens doors to stable careers and faster integration.

Internal Medicine, Family Medicine, Psychiatry, and Pediatrics remain consistently welcoming to IMGs, while highly competitive surgical and subspecialty fields continue to pose significant barriers despite prior practice.

Ultimately, success lies in aligning long-term goals with realistic opportunities, reframing your narrative, and demonstrating both humility and confidence. By tailoring your application thoughtfully, you can transform your international background into a strength and secure a place in the U.S. medical system.

Chapter 13: Leveraging International Experience in the Residency Match

For International Medical Graduates who have already completed their medical training and, in many cases, years of independent practice abroad, entering the U.S. residency Match presents a unique set of challenges.

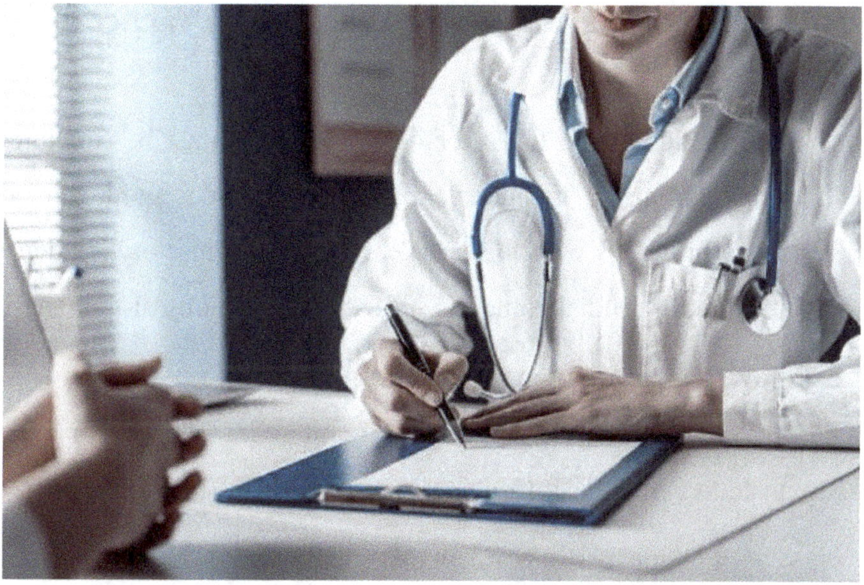

On one hand, IMGs often bring a depth of clinical experience, patient volume, and procedural knowledge that many U.S. graduates lack at the time of residency application. On the other hand, the residency Match system is designed to evaluate all candidates, whether a fresh graduate or a seasoned practitioner, on similar criteria: standardized exams, U.S. clinical experience, letters of recommendation, and interview performance.

This chapter explores how experienced international physicians can translate their background into a competitive application while avoiding common pitfalls, such as appearing overqualified or disconnected from the U.S. system. The goal is not to minimize past achievements, but to frame them in a way that highlights adaptability, humility, and readiness to learn again.

How to Translate Years of International Practice into a U.S.-Friendly CV

A curriculum vitae (CV) for U.S. residency must be structured differently from a traditional physician résumé used abroad. Residency programs want to see a clear academic trajectory, evidence of clinical skills, and alignment with U.S. expectations of training.

1. Prioritize Relevance to U.S. Programs

Many IMGs mistakenly list every conference attended or every administrative role held, resulting in a bloated CV. Instead:

- Highlight clinical roles that demonstrate depth (such as *"Managed daily inpatient census of 20 to 30 patients, including acute care management, chronic disease control, and interdisciplinary team coordination"*).
- Focus on academic contributions (teaching medical students, supervising interns, publishing).

- Limit less relevant items, such as local community awards, unless they reflect transferable skills (leadership, service, patient advocacy).

2. Standardize Terminology

Residency program directors may not understand terms like *"Senior Registrar," "House Officer,"* or *"Consultant."* Translate them into U.S.-equivalent language:

- *"Attending physician" → "Independent practitioner"*
- *"Registrar" → "Resident-level physician"*
- *"House Officer" → "Intern-equivalent role"*

This ensures clarity and avoids assumptions about inflated titles.

3. Quantify Experience

Numbers stand out in a CV. Instead of *"Performed obstetric procedures,"* write:

- *"Delivered over 1,200 babies over a seven-year period, including high-risk vaginal deliveries and cesarean sections."*
- *"Performed approximately 300 endoscopies, with independent responsibility for pre- and post-procedure care."*

Quantification allows U.S. reviewers to quickly gauge the breadth and depth of your practice.

4. Integrate Research and Teaching

Even if your primary role was clinical, U.S. programs value evidence of scholarship:

- List research projects, even local or non-indexed ones, framed as contributions to evidence-based care.
- Highlight teaching experience (lectures, bedside teaching, mentorship of junior doctors).
- Use verbs such as *organized, designed, developed,* and *supervised* to show leadership in academic contributions.

Framing Patient Volume, Procedures, and Teaching Experience in ERAS Applications

The Electronic Residency Application Service (ERAS) is where your experiences are distilled into structured entries. Here, framing is everything.

1. Clinical Experience Entries

Avoid vague descriptions. Instead of *"Worked as a physician in general practice,"* use:

"Provided primary and acute care to a diverse patient panel of approximately 4,000 individuals, managing high patient volume (30 to 40 visits per day) across internal medicine, pediatrics, and obstetrics."

This style demonstrates scope of practice, adaptability, and efficiency.

2. Procedural Skills

Residency programs want residents who are technically capable but not set in their ways. Frame procedures as breadth of exposure, not final mastery:

- *"Performed over 200 lumbar punctures independently, with focus on diagnostic yield and infection prevention protocols."*
- *"Assisted in over 300 orthopedic surgeries, including trauma stabilization, fracture fixation, and arthroplasty."*

3. Teaching Experience

Residency inherently involves teaching. U.S. programs view prior teaching as a positive predictor of leadership:

- *"Developed and delivered a weekly clinical case conference for 20 medical students, emphasizing problem-based learning."*
- *"Supervised 10 junior residents annually, providing bedside instruction, case review, and procedural guidance."*

Crafting a Personal Statement that Honors Past Achievements without Appearing "Overqualified"

The personal statement is where many experienced IMGs inadvertently undermine themselves. If framed incorrectly, it may suggest that you see residency as a step backward, or worse, as beneath your prior achievements.

1. Honor the Past, Emphasize the Future

Structure your statement to:

- Briefly acknowledge past accomplishments.
- Emphasize your desire to adapt to U.S. standards and continue lifelong learning.
- Demonstrate enthusiasm for training, not entitlement to a position.

2. Avoid Common Pitfalls

- **Overqualification trap:** Statements like *"After 20 years of independent practice, I now seek U.S. training"* may backfire. Instead:
- *"My years in practice deepened my clinical judgment, but I seek U.S. training to align my skills with American standards of patient care."*
- **Negative comparisons:** Never contrast U.S. training unfavorably with your home system. Focus on what draws you to the U.S. system, such as team-based care, research integration, or advanced technology.

3. Showcase Adaptability

Residency programs need reassurance that you will accept supervision and feedback. Include examples of learning from colleagues, adapting to new systems, or embracing innovation in your prior work.

The Fine Balance Between Emphasizing Leadership vs. Showing Readiness to Train Again

Residency programs value leadership but must be convinced that you are willing to function in a trainee role. Striking this balance requires careful framing.

1. When to Highlight Leadership

- When describing teaching roles, committee membership, or public health projects.
- When showing initiative, such as implementing new protocols or leading research.

2. When to Show Humility

- Acknowledge that medicine is constantly evolving and that U.S. residency offers access to updated technologies and evidence-based approaches.
- Show excitement for structured mentorship and multidisciplinary teamwork, even if you were previously in charge.

Example Statement:

"While I previously supervised junior doctors in my home country, I am eager to now be on the learning side of structured supervision, where I can refine my clinical skills under guidance while also contributing my experience in teaching and teamwork."

This balance reassures programs that you will be a team player, not a disruptive presence.

Strong Letters of Recommendation from International vs. U.S. Mentors , How to Position Both

Letters of recommendation (LoRs) are among the most influential elements of a residency application. For IMGs, the challenge lies in balancing letters from home-country mentors with U.S. references.

1. U.S. Letters Carry More Weight

Residency programs often prioritize LoRs from U.S. physicians because they demonstrate:

- Direct observation of your clinical performance in the U.S. healthcare setting.
- Familiarity with the expectations of U.S. residency training.
- Standardized language (most U.S. physicians know how to write residency LoRs).

Tip: Aim for at least two to three U.S. letters, ideally from clinical rotations, observerships, or research collaborations.

2. Value of International Letters

Strong international LoRs are not useless, especially if:

- They come from a highly regarded physician or professor.
- They speak to your long-term professionalism, work ethic, and character.

- They document depth of clinical exposure (for example: *"Dr. X managed over 500 cardiology inpatients annually under my supervision."*)

3. Positioning Both Together

- Use U.S. letters to validate your readiness for the American system.
- Use international letters to underscore your depth of experience and character.
- Together, they provide a complete picture: competence abroad **and** adaptability in the U.S.

Sample Narratives of Successful Applications

To illustrate these strategies, here are fictionalized but realistic narratives of IMGs who leveraged their experience successfully.

Case 1: Dr. Ananya Patel , India → Internal Medicine

Dr. Patel practiced as an internist in Mumbai for six years. Initially, she worried her independent practice would make her appear overqualified. In her CV, she quantified her patient load (*"20 to 25 daily outpatients, 10 inpatients under continuous management"*) and highlighted teaching medical interns.

Her personal statement acknowledged her Indian practice but pivoted to her desire for structured research exposure in the U.S. She secured two U.S. letters from observerships and one from her department head in India.

During interviews, she emphasized adaptability: *"Although I was previously independent, I value the chance to refine my skills under supervision to ensure I meet U.S. standards."* She matched into Internal Medicine at a mid-sized university program.

Case 2: Dr. Chukwuemeka Okafor , Nigeria → Psychiatry

Dr. Okafor worked as a general physician in Lagos, with extensive exposure to psychiatric comorbidities. In ERAS, he framed this experience as broad patient care involving both physical and mental health challenges. He described running a weekly counseling group for patients with depression and HIV.

His personal statement highlighted his passion for mental health advocacy rather than medical independence alone. With one U.S. LoR from a psychiatry observership and two Nigerian references, he matched into Psychiatry.

Case 3: Dr. Maria Gonzalez , Colombia → Family Medicine

Dr. Gonzalez had eight years of family practice experience in rural Colombia. She emphasized her procedural versatility (deliveries, minor surgeries, preventive care) and community service.

In her CV, she quantified her work: *"Cared for a panel of 5,000 patients across all age groups."*

Her U.S. mentor from a family medicine observership wrote that she was *"remarkably adaptable, approaching U.S. clinical norms with humility despite her extensive experience."* She matched into

Family Medicine in the Midwest, where her bilingual skills became a major asset.

Conclusion

For IMGs with years of practice abroad, the residency Match is not simply a test of competence, but of adaptability, humility, and strategic communication.

Your background can be a strength if presented correctly:

- Translate experience into quantifiable, U.S.-friendly language.
- Frame achievements as preparation for structured training, not substitutes for it.
- Balance leadership with readiness to learn.
- Secure both U.S. and international letters to validate competence and character.
- Use your personal statement to show commitment, not entitlement.

Residency programs value maturity, perspective, and dedication. By carefully framing your international experience, you can transform what might seem like a mismatch into a compelling advantage, demonstrating that you are not only ready to train in the U.S., but also to enrich the learning environment with your unique journey.

Chapter 14:
Life After Residency for Experienced IMGs

Completing residency in the United States is a transformative milestone for International Medical Graduates. For many, it represents the culmination of years of sacrifice: leaving established practices, enduring a competitive Match process, repeating training, and adjusting to a new professional hierarchy.

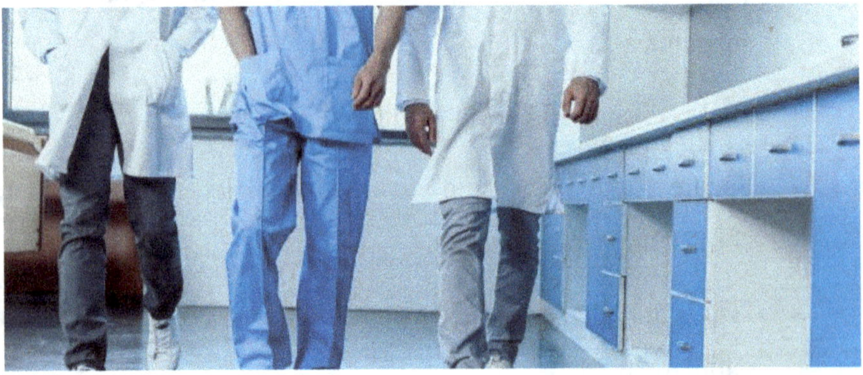

Yet, residency is not the end of the journey, it is the beginning of a new chapter as a fully licensed physician in the U.S.

For experienced IMGs, post-residency life brings unique opportunities and challenges. Unlike U.S. medical graduates, IMGs often carry the perspective of having already been independent practitioners abroad. This background, combined with U.S. training, creates a dual professional identity that can be leveraged in leadership, education, underserved medicine, global health, and academic careers.

At the same time, issues such as financial rebuilding, immigration status, and redefining one's identity must be carefully navigated.

This chapter explores life after residency for experienced IMGs and provides a roadmap for maximizing opportunities, addressing challenges, and shaping a long-term career.

Career Advancement Opportunities: Leadership, Education, and Research

Once residency is complete, IMGs transition from supervised trainees to independent attending physicians. This opens doors for advancement beyond clinical practice.

1. Leadership Roles in Healthcare Systems

Many IMGs who held leadership responsibilities abroad naturally gravitate toward positions of influence in the U.S. healthcare system. Opportunities include:

- **Medical Directorships:** Overseeing a clinic, hospital unit, or specialty service line. Responsibilities may involve quality improvement, patient safety, and staff coordination.
- **Department or Division Leadership:** Academic centers often seek physicians with diverse experiences to lead clinical services or training programs.

- **Administrative Leadership:** Physicians with strong organizational skills may become Chief Medical Officers (CMOs) or hold roles in hospital administration.

For IMGs, leadership roles require careful navigation. While prior leadership abroad demonstrates capability, U.S. healthcare leadership demands familiarity with regulatory standards, billing practices, and cultural expectations.

Enrolling in leadership training programs, such as those offered by the American Association for Physician Leadership (AAPL), or completing an MBA in Healthcare Management can accelerate this trajectory.

2. Roles in Medical Education

Residency programs value physicians with teaching experience. IMGs who previously supervised medical students and interns abroad can build on this foundation by:

- Becoming core faculty in residency programs.
- Serving as Clerkship Directors or Residency Program Directors.
- Teaching in medical schools as clinical professors.

U.S. institutions increasingly emphasize diversity and global health perspectives, making IMG educators especially valuable. Those who invest in education-focused fellowships (such as Medical Education Fellowships) or pursue a Master of Health Professions Education (MHPE) can advance rapidly in this field.

3. Opportunities in Research

Experienced IMGs often bring a clinically grounded perspective shaped by years of practice abroad. This can translate into innovative research questions.

Post-residency options include:

- Clinical trials, especially in diverse or underserved populations.
- Health disparities research, where dual international and U.S. perspectives are invaluable.
- Collaborations with global health institutions, NGOs, and universities.

Pursuing fellowships with research components (for example, cardiology, oncology, or infectious diseases) or seeking grants through the National Institutes of Health (NIH) or private foundations can position IMGs as physician-researchers.

Using Dual Experience as an Advantage

One of the most underappreciated assets IMGs bring is their dual clinical experience. Having treated patients abroad and trained in the U.S. makes them uniquely equipped for certain roles.

1. Serving Underserved Areas in the U.S.

Residency programs and state governments actively encourage physicians to work in rural and underserved communities. IMGs, accustomed to resource-limited environments abroad, often excel in these roles.

- Programs such as the National Health Service Corps (NHSC) offer loan repayment for service in shortage areas.
- Hospitals in rural regions may provide incentives such as higher salaries, signing bonuses, or relocation packages.

IMGs can leverage their adaptability and resilience from practicing abroad to thrive in these environments, often gaining rapid promotion opportunities.

2. Global Health and International Partnerships

Having practiced abroad, IMGs are natural fits for global health initiatives. Career paths include:

- Academic centers with global health divisions.
- NGOs and international agencies (such as the WHO or Médecins Sans Frontières).
- U.S. institutions establishing overseas partnerships.

For example, an IMG who practiced in sub-Saharan Africa before U.S. training might spearhead global health electives for U.S. residents or collaborate on research addressing tropical diseases.

3. Academic Medicine

U.S. academic centers increasingly value diverse experiences. IMGs who combine international practice with U.S. residency can become thought leaders in:

- Cross-cultural patient care.
- Comparative healthcare systems.
- Innovations in training international residents or fellows.

Publishing scholarly work that draws on both backgrounds, such as outcomes across different systems or strategies for immigrant patient populations, can create a distinct academic niche.

Financial Considerations: Rebuilding Income After Residency

For many IMGs, residency represents years of financial sacrifice. Unlike U.S. graduates who are just beginning their earning potential, experienced IMGs often face the reality of a significant financial step-down during training. Post-residency, financial recovery becomes a priority.

1. Transition from Resident to Attending Income

- Residency salaries typically range from $55,000 to $70,000 annually.
- Attending salaries, depending on specialty, location, and setting, can range from $180,000 in primary care to $500,000 or more in surgical fields.

This dramatic increase allows IMGs to catch up on financial goals, paying off debts, supporting families, and saving for retirement.

2. Managing Debt and Obligations

While IMGs may not carry U.S. medical school debt, they often face:

- Relocation expenses.
- Licensing and examination fees.
- Family support costs, especially if dependents remain abroad.

Key strategies include:

- Early investment in retirement accounts (401(k), IRA).
- Consulting financial advisors experienced in physician finance.
- Exploring loan repayment or incentive programs tied to underserved service.

3. Strategic Career Choices for Financial Growth

IMGs can accelerate financial recovery by:

- Choosing higher-paying geographic regions, often rural or underserved.
- Negotiating contracts with careful attention to bonuses, benefits, and malpractice coverage.
- Considering locum tenens work to supplement income while exploring long-term positions.

Immigration Pathways: From J-1 Waiver to Permanent Residency and Citizenship

Immigration remains one of the most defining aspects of an IMG's career trajectory in the U.S. While medical training provides a pathway, navigating visas and residency status is complex.

1. J-1 Visa Waiver Options

Most IMGs train on a J-1 exchange visitor visa, which requires a two-year home-country return unless a waiver is obtained. Options include:

- **Conrad 30 Waiver Program:** Allows each U.S. state to sponsor up to 30 physicians annually to work in underserved areas for three years.
- **Federal Programs:** Agencies such as the Veterans Health Administration or the Department of Health and Human Services may also sponsor waivers.

2. H-1B Visa for Physicians

Some IMGs enter residency on an H-1B visa. Advantages include:

- No two-year home return requirement.
- Direct transition to employment-based green card pathways.

However, H-1B visas are cap-subject, making them more difficult to obtain.

3. Transition to Permanent Residency (Green Card)

After completing a J-1 waiver service commitment or securing H-1B sponsorship, many IMGs pursue permanent residency through:

- Employment-based sponsorship, including EB-2 National Interest Waivers for physicians working in underserved areas.
- Employer-sponsored green cards, typically through large health systems.

4. Path to Citizenship

Permanent residents may apply for U.S. citizenship after five years. Citizenship provides stability, freedom from visa renewals, and expanded opportunities in leadership and government-affiliated roles.

Long-Term Identity: Blending "Former Physician Abroad" and "U.S.-Trained Physician"

Perhaps the most profound challenge for experienced IMGs is identity integration. After years of independent practice abroad followed by supervised training in the U.S., IMGs must reconcile two professional selves.

1. Overcoming the "Step Backward" Narrative

Residency may feel like regression, but reframing is essential:

- View U.S. residency as adaptation, not demotion.
- Recognize that U.S. training provides a globally recognized credential, enabling practice worldwide.

2. Embracing a Dual Identity

Successful IMGs often embrace a blended identity:

- **Former physician abroad:** Bringing resilience, resourcefulness, and cultural sensitivity.
- **U.S.-trained physician:** Demonstrating mastery of advanced systems, protocols, and technology.

This dual perspective enhances clinical care, enriches teaching, and expands leadership potential.

3. Giving Back

Many IMGs eventually bridge systems by:

- Training the next generation of IMGs.
- Establishing exchange programs between home-country institutions and U.S. centers.
- Engaging in diaspora networks to improve healthcare globally.

4. Personal Fulfillment

Identity is not only professional but personal. For many IMGs, building a career in the U.S. means creating a new home, balancing heritage with integration, and legacy with innovation.

Case Snapshots: IMGs After Residency

Case 1: Dr. Hassan – From Egypt to U.S. Hospital Leadership: After practicing as a cardiologist in Cairo, Dr. Hassan completed a U.S. internal medicine residency followed by a cardiology fellowship. He leveraged his dual experience to become a department chair at a major teaching hospital, emphasizing diversity in leadership.

Case 2: Dr. Rivera – From Peru to Rural Family Medicine: Dr. Rivera, who once ran a family clinic in Lima, accepted a Conrad 30 waiver position in rural Kansas. Her adaptability in resource-limited environments made her a community leader, and she later directed a residency program to mentor new IMGs.

Case 3: Dr. Chen – From China to Academic Researcher: Dr. Chen's background in infectious diseases research abroad, combined with U.S. residency training, propelled him into an NIH-funded laboratory, where he leads studies on emerging pathogens. His career demonstrates the research potential of dual training.

Conclusion

Life after residency for experienced IMGs is both liberating and demanding. The challenges, financial recovery, immigration navigation, and identity integration, are real. But so are the opportunities: leadership, education, research, underserved medicine, and global health.

By leveraging both their international roots and U.S. training, IMGs can carve out unique, impactful careers. Rather than viewing their journey as one of loss or duplication, successful IMGs embrace it as a fusion of strengths, shaping them into global physicians uniquely prepared to meet the challenges of modern medicine.

Conclusion: Your Roadmap to Success

As we come to the close of this journey through the many layers of becoming a physician in the United States, it is worth pausing to reflect not only on the information presented but also on what it truly means for you, as an international medical graduate, a medical student, or a practicing physician abroad who is considering, or already walking, the U.S. path.

This book was never meant to be simply a technical guide. It was written to serve as both a roadmap and a companion, one that reminds you that the process, while demanding, is navigable and deeply rewarding. For every statistic about competitiveness, every discussion of visas or applications, there are countless untold stories of IMGs who have walked the same path, faced the same uncertainty, and emerged not only as successful physicians in the U.S. but also as leaders, mentors, and innovators in global healthcare.

Recapping the Journey

We began with a broad overview of the U.S. medical system, outlining how it differs from international structures and how you, as an IMG, fit into that framework. Understanding accreditation bodies, patient-centered care, and interprofessional collaboration was the first step in grasping the ecosystem you are about to enter.

From there, we explored the preparatory phase before even setting foot in the U.S. This meant gathering credentials, navigating visas, and making thoughtful choices about whether the U.S. is the right destination for you. For many, this stage is where resilience is first tested, when you must balance logistics, paperwork, and uncertainty with the hope of a new career horizon.

Once in the U.S., we moved through the practical realities of settling into life: housing, banking, cultural adaptation, and building a support system. These details may seem small, but they can be the difference between thriving and feeling overwhelmed in a new country. Alongside these adjustments, we tackled the academic cornerstone of your U.S. medical journey: the USMLE examinations. Here, we emphasized not just study strategies and resources, but also the emotional perseverance required to balance financial, personal, and professional demands.

The middle chapters guided you through the vital building blocks of your U.S. profile, clinical experience, research opportunities, and letters of recommendation. These are the spaces where you demonstrate your adaptability, competence, and value to the U.S. healthcare system. Whether through observerships, externships, or publications, you are weaving a narrative that shows you are not only capable but uniquely positioned to contribute.

From there, the focus shifted to the residency application process, interviews, and ultimately, life in residency itself. These stages test not just your academic preparation but also your resilience, humility, and interpersonal skills. We examined common challenges such as impostor syndrome, stress, and the steep learning curve of adapting to U.S. residency life.

Finally, the latter chapters spoke directly to practicing physicians who face the difficult but empowering transition of moving from independent practice abroad to supervised training in the U.S. This is where humility meets strength, where years of experience can feel overshadowed by the title of "trainee," yet where new opportunities for growth, reinvention, and impact unfold.

Throughout, we looked beyond residency, toward fellowships, independent practice, leadership roles, and long-term identity as a globally trained physician who bridges two worlds.

The Core Message: Resilience and Persistence Pay Off

Across all stages of this roadmap, one truth stands out: resilience and persistence are the defining traits of successful IMGs. The challenges are real, visa restrictions, financial strain, cultural barriers, competitive examinations, and the emotional weight of starting again in a new system.

Yet, history is filled with IMGs who have overcome these very obstacles. They have become respected attending physicians, academic leaders, program directors, and policy advocates who shape healthcare in the U.S. and beyond.

What separates those who succeed is not merely intelligence or resources, but the ability to persist when progress feels slow, to remain adaptable when setbacks occur, and to continually learn from each stage of the journey.

Embracing Diversity and Global Contribution

As an IMG, you carry something invaluable into the U.S. system: perspective. You represent the diversity of global medicine, the thousands of hours spent treating patients in rural villages, bustling urban hospitals, or underserved clinics abroad. You bring with you resilience born from resourcefulness, cultural sensitivity honed from caring for diverse populations, and a perspective that enriches the increasingly multicultural fabric of U.S. healthcare.

Far from being a disadvantage, your background is your strength. It allows you to connect with immigrant patients who might otherwise feel misunderstood, to introduce innovative approaches learned abroad, and to embody the principle that medicine is truly a global calling. In a healthcare landscape that increasingly values inclusivity and cultural competence, your role as an IMG is not supplementary, it is essential.

Practical Next Steps

As you close this book, consider the following action points to anchor your next phase:

1. **Revisit your "why."** Before diving back into applications, examinations, or paperwork, remind yourself why you chose this journey. Anchoring in purpose fuels persistence.

2. **Map your timeline.** Break your roadmap into stages, credentialing, exams, clinical experience, applications. Assign realistic timelines while allowing flexibility for unexpected detours.
3. **Invest in community.** Seek mentorship, join IMG networks, and build a support system. The journey is too long and challenging to walk alone.
4. **Balance ambition with self-care.** Success is not achieved by burnout. Build habits, exercise, mindfulness, hobbies, that sustain resilience.
5. **Stay informed.** The U.S. medical landscape evolves. Regularly consult ECFMG, NRMP, and specialty organizations for updates.
6. **Celebrate small wins.** Passing Step 1, securing an observership, submitting your ERAS application, each milestone deserves recognition.

Looking Ahead

Your path may be long, but it is also extraordinary. Few professions demand the same blend of intellect, resilience, and compassion as medicine, and few journeys test those qualities as thoroughly as the IMG path to U.S. practice.

If you persevere, you will not only achieve the personal dream of becoming a U.S. physician but also join a lineage of doctors who have expanded what is possible in global healthcare.

Success is not measured solely by matching into the most competitive specialty or training at the most prestigious institution. Success lies in becoming the kind of physician who serves patients with skill, empathy, and integrity, whether in a bustling academic center, a community hospital, or an underserved rural clinic.

The United States needs you. Patients need you. And the future of medicine benefits from your voice, your expertise, and your unique story.

Final Encouragement

If there is one message to take from this book, let it be this: your journey is not only possible, it is worth it. Every sleepless night of studying, every form completed, every rejection transformed into resilience contributes to shaping you into a stronger physician and a deeper human being.

Medicine is a calling, not merely a career. Your calling has already carried you across continents, languages, and systems. As you take your next steps, walk with confidence, knowing that you are prepared, capable, and needed.

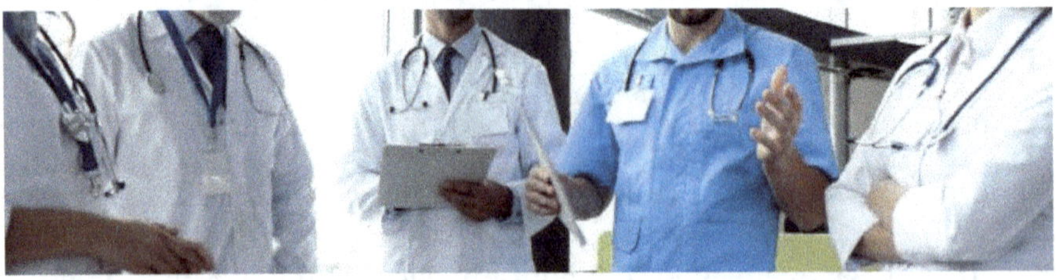

This roadmap is yours now. Follow it with courage, adapt it with wisdom, and remember, you are not just pursuing a medical career in the U.S. You are building a legacy of global healing.

Wish you good luck!

Appendices & Resources

Glossary of Key Terms

The world of U.S. medical training comes with its own vocabulary. Below is a glossary of the most frequently used terms you will encounter as an IMG.

- **ACGME (Accreditation Council for Graduate Medical Education):** The body responsible for accrediting residency and fellowship programs in the U.S.
- **AMGs (American Medical Graduates):** Medical graduates from U.S. or Canadian medical schools.
- **ECFMG (Educational Commission for Foreign Medical Graduates):** The organization that certifies international medical graduates to enter U.S. residency programs.
- **ERAS (Electronic Residency Application Service):** The centralized system used to apply to residency and fellowship programs.
- **IMG (International Medical Graduate):** A physician who earned their medical degree outside the U.S. or Canada.
- **LCME (Liaison Committee on Medical Education):** Accrediting body for medical schools in the U.S. and Canada.
- **LOR (Letter of Recommendation):** A document written by a physician or mentor recommending you for residency, usually highlighting your clinical skills, professionalism, and character.

- **Match:** Short for "The Match," the annual system that places applicants into residency programs through the NRMP.
- **MSPE (Medical Student Performance Evaluation):** Also known as the Dean's Letter; summarizes your academic performance.
- **NBME (National Board of Medical Examiners):** The organization that co-develops the USMLE examinations.
- **NRMP (National Resident Matching Program):** The organization that runs "The Match."
- **Observership:** A type of U.S. clinical experience where IMGs shadow physicians without direct patient care responsibilities.
- **Residency:** Graduate medical education training following medical school, typically 3 to 7 years depending on specialty.
- **SOAP (Supplemental Offer and Acceptance Program):** A process for unmatched applicants to obtain unfilled residency positions after Match Day.
- **Step Exams (USMLE):** Licensing exams required for medical licensure and residency applications, including Step 1, Step 2 CK, and Step 3.
- **USCE (U.S. Clinical Experience):** Clinical exposure in the U.S. through observerships, externships, electives, or clerkships.

- **Visa (J-1, H-1B):** Work authorization categories that determine how IMGs train and practice in the U.S.

Timeline Planner for IMGs

Every IMG's journey is unique, but having a structured timeline is crucial to staying organized and avoiding delays. Below is a suggested 4- to 5-year roadmap from preparation to independent practice.

Year 1: Early Preparation

- Research destination countries (U.S., Canada, UK, Australia).
- Begin credential evaluation (WES, ECFMG).
- Collect transcripts, diplomas, and LORs from your home country.
- Register for TOEFL/IELTS if required.
- Start preparing for USMLE Step 1.

Year 2: Testing and Early Experience

- Sit for Step 1.
- Begin Step 2 CK preparation.
- Explore short-term research opportunities or observerships in the U.S.
- Network with mentors, IMG alumni, and professional societies.
- Budget and arrange finances for examinations and travel.

Year 3: Clinical Experience and Application Preparation

- Complete Step 2 CK.
- Secure U.S. clinical experience (observerships, externships, clerkships).
- Begin drafting your personal statement and CV.
- Request U.S.-based letters of recommendation.
- Research residency programs, specialty competitiveness, and visa policies.
- Register with ERAS (June).

Year 4: Residency Applications

- Submit ERAS applications in September.
- Prepare thoroughly for interviews (mock interviews, practice questions).
- Attend interviews (October–January).
- Participate in The Match (rank order list due in February).
- If unmatched, prepare for SOAP in March.

Year 5 and Beyond: Residency and Career Planning

- Start residency in July.
- Take Step 3 (usually during residency year 1 or 2).
- Plan for fellowships or independent practice.
- If on a J-1 visa, explore waiver programs for underserved areas.

Tip: Adjust this timeline based on personal pace. Some IMGs may complete the process in 2 to 3 years, while others may require 5 to 6 years depending on finances, family responsibilities, or prior commitments.

Useful Websites, Organizations, and Support Groups

Having reliable resources at your fingertips can make this journey smoother. Below is a curated list.

Official Organizations

- **ECFMG:** www.ecfmg.org – Certification and credential verification for IMGs.
- **USMLE:** www.usmle.org – Official information about licensing examinations.
- **NRMP:** www.nrmp.org – Match and SOAP details.
- **ERAS/AAMC:** students-residents.aamc.org – Residency application system and resources.
- **FSMB (Federation of State Medical Boards):** www.fsmb.org – State licensure information.

Study and Exam Preparation

- **UWorld:** www.uworld.com – Premier USMLE practice question bank.
- **NBME:** www.nbme.org – Self-assessments and practice examinations.

- **First Aid for the USMLE:** Widely used study guide (book and online resources).

IMG-Specific Networks

- **AMA IMG Section:** www.ama-assn.org – Advocacy and professional support.
- **Match A Resident:** www.matcharesident.com – Residency program research for IMGs.
- **Physician Moms Group (Facebook):** Support for female physicians balancing career and family.
- **Reddit r/IMGreddit:** Peer-to-peer advice and shared experiences.

Support and Mentorship

- **Doctors Without Borders (MSF):** Opportunities for global health involvement.
- **Society of Hospital Medicine (SHM):** Networking for IMGs in Internal Medicine.
- **Local alumni associations:** Indian Medical Association of North America, Nigerian Doctors in the U.S., and similar groups.

Sample Personal Statement

Note: This is an illustrative sample. Do not copy; instead, use it to structure your own authentic narrative.

Personal Statement Example (Internal Medicine):

Growing up in India, I saw firsthand the challenges patients face in rural communities with limited access to healthcare. During my clinical rotations at [University Hospital], I was drawn to Internal Medicine because it allowed me to integrate knowledge across specialties while forming long-term relationships with patients.

My U.S. clinical experience at [XYZ Medical Center] reinforced my interest. I learned to adapt quickly to electronic medical record systems, participate in team-based rounds, and communicate effectively with diverse patient populations. I particularly valued my mentor's feedback that I "demonstrated humility and eagerness to learn," qualities I carry with me daily.

Beyond clinical care, I am passionate about preventive medicine and research. My project on diabetes outcomes in underserved populations was presented as a poster at the [ABC Conference], deepening my commitment to addressing healthcare disparities.

As an IMG, I bring the resilience developed in resource-limited settings, cultural competence across diverse patient populations, and a commitment to lifelong learning. I look forward to joining a residency program where I can grow as a clinician, contribute to research, and serve both local and global communities.

Sample Curriculum Vitae (CV)

Name, MD

Email | Phone | Address | LinkedIn

Education

- MBBS, University of Mumbai – Graduated 2018
- ECFMG Certification – 2022

Licensure / Examinations

- USMLE Step 1: Passed (245)
- USMLE Step 2 CK: Passed (250)
- Step 3: Scheduled for 2023

Clinical Experience

- **Externship – XYZ Medical Center, New York, NY** Observed and assisted in Internal Medicine ward rounds; conducted patient histories and physical examinations under supervision.
- **Observership – ABC Hospital, Houston, TX** Shadowed attending physicians in Cardiology; participated in case discussions and journal clubs.

Research

- Diabetes Outcomes in Underserved Communities – Poster presentation at ABC Conference, 2021.

- Co-author, *Journal of Global Health Research* – Article on infectious disease management in rural India, 2020.

Publications

- [List peer-reviewed articles, posters, and abstracts if applicable.]

Leadership and Volunteering

- President, Medical Student Association, University of Mumbai.
- Volunteer Physician, Rural Health Camp, Maharashtra (2019).

Skills

- Languages: English, Hindi, Marathi.
- Electronic Medical Record (EMR) systems: Epic, Cerner.

Final Note on Resources

These appendices are not meant to be exhaustive, but rather a practical toolkit. With a glossary to demystify terminology, a structured timeline to guide your steps, trusted organizations to rely on, and samples to model your applications, you now have essential building blocks for the journey ahead.

The rest comes from tailoring these tools to your unique path, staying consistent, and drawing strength from the community of IMGs who came before you.

www.ingramcontent.com/pod-product-compliance
Lightning Source LLC
LaVergne TN
LVHW052256200926
848481LV00002B/386